WITHDRAWN FROM STOCK
The University of Liverpool

Please return or
below. A fine is
Books may be rec
another reader.
Recall, books m
5412.

DUE TO RETURN
3 0 APR 1996

CANCELLED

DUE FOR RETURN
27 MAY 1997

CANCELLED

For conditions c

THE ELECTRICAL ACTIVITY
OF THE NERVOUS SYSTEM

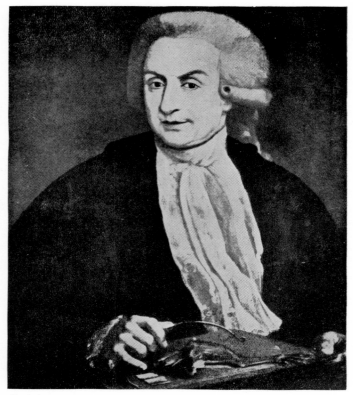

Luigi Galvani (1737–1798)

(From an oil-painting in the Library of the University of Bologna, reproduced by courtesy of Dr. Giulio Pupilli)

THE
ELECTRICAL ACTIVITY
OF THE
NERVOUS SYSTEM

A Textbook for Students

BY

MARY A. B. BRAZIER
B.Sc., Ph.D., D.Sc. (London)

Brain Research Institute
University of California, Los Angeles

THIRD EDITION

LONDON
Pitman Medical Publishing Co. Ltd

First published 1951
Revised and reprinted 1953
Reprinted 1958
Second edition 1960
Reprinted 1961
Reprinted 1966
Third edition 1968

PITMAN MEDICAL PUBLISHING COMPANY Lᴛᴅ
46 CHARLOTTE STREET, LONDON, W1

ASSOCIATED COMPANIES

SIR ISAAC PITMAN & SONS Lᴛᴅ
PITMAN HOUSE, PARKER STREET, KINGSWAY, LONDON, WC2
THE PITMAN PRESS, BATH
PITMAN HOUSE, BOUVERIE STREET, CARLTON, VICTORIA 3053
P.O. BOX 7721, JOHANNESBURG, TRANSVAAL
P.O. BOX 6038, PORTAL STREET, NAIROBI

PITMAN PUBLISHING CORPORATION
20 EAST 46TH STREET, NEW YORK, N.Y. 10017

SIR ISAAC PITMAN (CANADA) Lᴛᴅ
PITMAN HOUSE, 381–383 CHURCH STREET, TORONTO

SBN: 272 75448 X

MADE IN GREAT BRITAIN AT THE PITMAN PRESS, BATH

Note

THIS book is written for students with the purpose of bringing together under one cover a survey of the electrical activity of the nervous system. Those who want to go farther will find signposts to the primary sources in the list of references at the end of each section. As this is a textbook intended for the English-speaking student, references in other languages have been kept to a minimum.

This is not intended to be a technical manual. Technical methods are constantly changing with the development of instrumental design, and would no sooner be written down than superseded. But even if this were not so, the only place to learn technique is in the laboratory.

M.A.B.B.

Preface to the Second Edition

SOME major changes in the science of neurophysiology have developed in the nine years since the first edition of this book was prepared. Outstanding among these is a growing realisation of great plasticity of the component mechanisms that are the elements of nervous activity. Freed at last from the binding rigidity of the all-or-nothing law by recognition that such restrictive behaviour is confined only to the conducting fibre, the subtle reactions of the nervous system become more understandable. Processes for achieving graded responses, at both the peripheral and the central ends of these conductors, permit a complexity of performance that would be denied to a solely digital system.

This knowledge has largely been contributed by those who work with microelectrodes. This first stage of their achievement was to report the current flows they found surrounding the individual cells of nervous tissue. From this they have progressed to recordings from within the substance of the nerve cells. It was as though at first the electrophysiologist were walking down a street, looking at the houses, peering at the closed windows, and inferring the behaviour of the inmates from the comings and goings through the doors. Now he has pushed the doors open and is beginning to report at first-hand the activity inside the rooms.

Of the pieces of knowledge that have derived from such studies one of the most basic is that the component parts of the individual neurone have different properties. The rate of discharge, the threshold for discharge, and the rate of repolarisation varying from one part of the membrane to another in the same neurone, provide mutually interacting variables, even at the unitary level.

At an integrative level the demonstration of centrifugal

vii

control, exerted by the central nervous system over the receptors in the periphery modulating the messages they send centralwards, is one of the advances that has great importance for any formulation that may be made about integration of nervous activity. The formerly accepted dichotomy between sensory and motor systems is no longer so valid, and a further degree of sophistication is called for in the stimulus-response concepts that have ruled for so long.

In the last nine years a wealth of new material bearing on the integration of neuronal activity has come from the recognition of the rôle that the reticular formation of the brain stem plays as an intermediary and modulator of sensory and motor activity through reciprocal interaction with the cortex, the cerebellum and the periphery. By the unfolding of knowledge of these systems a bridge can now be envisaged between physiologically-definable neuronal events and behavioural activity whose description has previously lain in another realm of discourse.

With the mastering of techniques for implanting electrodes in the nervous system, knowledge is slowly accumulating about nervous activity in unanaesthetised, unrestrained, freely-moving animals. We look at our shelves and realise that our textbooks teach us the pathological physiology of the anaesthetised or surgically-maimed animal, the morphological anatomy of the dead. The greater portion of this book has perforce to follow on these lines, for not yet have data from the physiological animal been gathered for more than a small portion of this great field. Perhaps in another nine years it may be possible for someone to give us a book on the electrical activity of the physiological nervous system.

MARY A. B. BRAZIER

MASSACHUSETTS GENERAL HOSPITAL
BOSTON
1958

Preface to the Third Edition

In the development of our knowledge about the electrical activity of the nervous system there are certain outstanding landmarks. Some, like the initial discovery in the nineteenth century of the electrical character of the nerve impulse and, in the early years of this century, the demonstration of the all-or-nothing character of its propagation, established the basic mechanism by which communication takes place in the nervous system. Other advances, such as the elucidation at mid-century of the existence and rôle of the non-specific ascending system of the brain stem, provided long-sought understanding of inter-actions at the highest levels of brain function, while in the same period, and at the other end of the scale, the intimate polarisation changes inside the nerve cell itself were first being success-fully explored, and a fuller realisation of the mechanisms by which the nervous system uses graded responses became possible.

In this second half of the twentieth century the biological sciences have benefitted from a tremendous technological achievement—the development of computers. Not since Loewenhoek, with his invention of the microscope, gave the biologist a powerful prosthesis for his vision has such power been added to his analytical techniques—a prosthesis aiding his cal-culating ability in both speed and complexity.

One would wish that the student of the nervous system would be familiar both with the work of the pioneers and with that of the *avant-garde* of this science, for let us not forget Santayana's warning that, 'those who cannot remember the past are condemned to repeat it'.

Mary A. B. Brazier

Brain Research Institute
University of California, Los Angeles
1966

Contents

Plates

In 1791 an article appeared in the Proceedings of the Bologna Academy reporting some experiments on frogs' legs which, it was claimed, proved the existence of animal electricity. This famous publication, 'De viribus electricitatis in motu musculari,' which started one of the great controversies of the time, was the work of the professor of anatomy at Bologna, Luigi Galvani. Volta's conviction that the electricity of Galvani's experiments derived from the presence of dissimilar metals led to the development of the Voltaic pile; Galvani's experiments led to the science of electrophysiology. His original treatise and the supplement to a tract published anonymously three years later ('Dell' arco conduttore'), which described muscle contraction in the absence of metals, were the foundations for the study of the electrical activity of the nervous system.

A Brief Outline of the Physiology of the Nervous System

AN understanding of the electrical activity of the nervous system requires a more detailed knowledge of its anatomy and physiology than can have space here, but a brief description will be outlined as a reminder of the principal structures involved, more detail being added in later chapters as the need arises.

The units of the nervous system of which the whole structure is composed are the nerve cells: bodies usually less than 1/10 mm in diameter and therefore just beyond the range of unaided vision. The microscope reveals the typical nerve cell as having three main parts: the cell body, the dendrites, and the axon or fibre which transmits excitation away from the cell body; all are parts of the cell proper and share a single nucleus. The knowledge that the nerve fibres with their multiple branches are actually protoplasmic outgrowths of the cell itself grew from the observation, made nearly a hundred years ago by Kölliker, that all fibres make direct connexions with cell bodies. The work of Ramón y Cajal gave the final proof. To avoid confusion between the cell body and the whole cell unit (including its fibres) the latter is usually spoken of as the neurone (Fig. 1).

All parts of the neurone are encased in a membrane which acts as a boundary between their chemical contents and those of the surrounding medium. Direct measurement of the electrical properties of the membrane in mammalian species was first established in the large motor neurones, where the resistivity was found to be of the order of 1000 ohms per cm^2 and the capacitance about 3μF/cm^2.

More modern techniques using intracellular microelectrodes have enabled investigators to measure the capacitance values for membranes of Betz cells in the neocortex of cats. The capacitances are found to be of the order of $2\mu F/cm^2$ and the resistivity about 4000 ohms per cm^2.

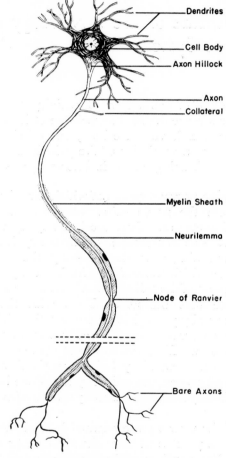

FIG. I. SCHEMATIC DRAWING OF A NERVE CELL

Some dimensions are grossly exaggerated for diagrammatic representation of the structures mentioned in the text.

In man and other mammals the fibres of the somatic nerves, that is, those which rapidly convey impulses from the sense organs to the brain and from the brain to the muscles to ensure immediate adjustment to the environment, are coated with a fatty sheath and are hence called medullated or myelinated nerves. The myelin of the sheath consists of regularly-arranged concentric rings of long lipoid molecules oriented tangentially. This structure can be clearly seen with polarised light through the ultramicroscope. In the sympathetic nervous system the post-ganglionic fibres have no apparent myelin sheath and the sensory fibres of the visceral nerves, which conduct with less speed, have only a thin coating of myelin or none at all. In addition to the axis cylinder, which is the main protoplasmic outgrowth from the cell body, there are many collaterals or threads branching off from the axon and forming intricate networks with neighbouring neurones. The nerve fibres of the peripheral nerves are encased in a nucleated sheath called the neurilemma. This is interrupted at intervals by constrictions known as the nodes of Ranvier. These structures were for long regarded as properties peculiar to peripheral nerves, but there is now evidence of somewhat similar node-like structures in the nerves of the central nervous system.

The highly schematised nerve cell shown in Fig. 1 more closely resembles the motor neurones of the spinal cord than any others of the nervous system. Nerve cells have a great diversity of form as may be seen from Bodian's illustration (reproduced as Fig. 2) in which the various neurone types are shown diagrammatically according to the degree of their connexion with other cells, those with the greatest wealth of interconnexion being shown at the top of the picture.

The chemical structure of the axoplasm (the protoplasm inside the axon) is being extensively investigated. It is a stiff gel containing a considerable amount of potassium, little sodium, chlorides and some protein. The ultrastructure of the cytoplasm of a neurone has been revealed by the electron microscope to contain Nissl bodies with mitochondria and fine filaments lying between them.

The human brain is constructed of many thousands of millions of these neurones, each cell communicating trans-synaptically with hundreds of others. There are great concentrations of these cells on the outside of the brain in the folded surface layer known as the cortex, and at the top of the brain stem in the basal ganglia, the subthalamic nuclei, the hypothalamus and the great cell masses of the thalamus. They constitute the grey matter, so called because of the appearance caused by the mass effect of millions of cells as seen by the naked eye. Most, but not all, of the axons are covered with a sheath of myelin which gives them a white appearance, whereas the cell-body and dendrites, having no myelin, appear grey in comparison.

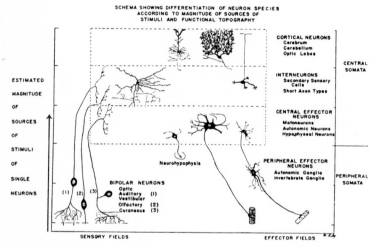

FIG. 2. THE GREAT DIVERSITY OF NEURONE TYPES FOUND IN THE MAMMALIAN NERVOUS SYSTEM

Here they are shown ranked according to the estimated number of other neurones bringing stimuli to them.

(From Bodian (1952) *Cold Spr. Harb. Symp. quant. Biol.*, **17**, 1.)

Neuroglia lies between the neurones and has important properties that reveal it to be of greater significance than a mere supportive tissue. The cerebellum with specialised cell bodies and fibre tracts lies below and behind the cerebrum with which it is intricately connected (Fig. 3).

The great tracts of nerve fibres running to and from the cells of the cortex can be classified in three main groups. The commissures are the fibres connecting the two hemispheres which cross from one side to the other, those from cortex to cortex mostly in the large band known as the corpus callosum. These are strictly speaking association fibres, but this name is usually reserved for those fibres which interconnect cortical areas in the same hemisphere. These run in the deeper part of the cortex or just below it and are far more numerous than any other type of neurone in the brain. The projection fibres are those which connect subcortical cell stations with the cortex. Many, but by no means all, afferent fibres reaching the cortex from below have their cell stations in the thalamus, whereas

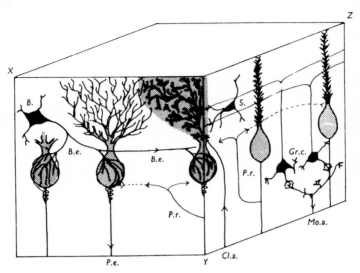

FIG. 3. SCHEMATIC REPRESENTATION OF CELLULAR
INTERCONNEXIONS IN THE CEREBELLAR CORTEX

Efferent paths (*P.e.*) from a Purkinje cell are shown to have recurrent collaterals (*P.r.*). Afferent connexions to the Purkinje cells come from the mossy fibres (*Mo.a.*) via the granular cells (*Gr.c.*), and from the climbing fibres (*Cl.a.*). Interconnexions with basket cells (*B.*) and Stellate cells (*S.*) form components of intracortical networks.

(From Granit and Phillips (1956) *J. Physiol.* (*Lond.*), **133**, 520.)

the axons of the cortical cells may end in the thalamus, brain stem or spinal cord.

The afferent fibres of the projection tracts emerge from their specific cell stations in the thalamus and fan out to the appropriate areas of the cortex (Fig. 4). These projection areas in the cortex are quite small in size but are arranged so that there is an approximate similarity of spatial pattern between the region of the body sending the message and the region of cortex receiving it. For example, the primary auditory cortex in the

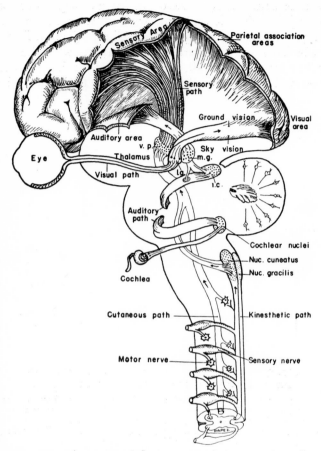

FIG. 4. THE FOUR MAIN SENSORY PATHWAYS TO THE CORTEX

The sensory path from the skin and the kinaesthetic path from the muscles both pass upward and through the thalamus (v.p.) and then continue to the sensory area of the post-central cortex. The auditory path from the cochlea passes through the cochlear nucleus, to the inferior colliculus, and to the medial geniculate body of the thalamus and thence to the auditory cortex of the temporal lobe. The visual path from the retina passes in the optic nerve to the lateral geniculate and thence to the visual area in the occipital cortex.

(From Papez (1948) *Human Growth and Development*. Cornell Co-operative Society.)

6

superior temporal gyrus receives its fibres in order of pitch; adjacent portions of the visual cortex near the calcarine fissure receive, in the same spatial pattern, fibres from adjacent portions of the retina; and the fibres conveying sense of muscle

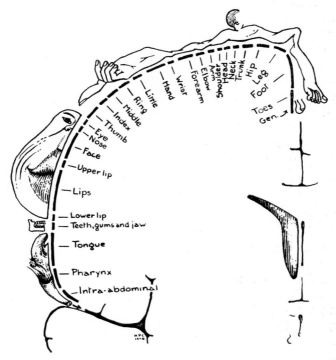

FIG. 5. SENSORY REPRESENTATION OF THE BODY IN THE
POSTCENTRAL GYRUS

This is a sensory homunculus designed by Penfield as a visualisation of the order and comparative size of representation of each part of the body in the postcentral gyrus from inside the longitudinal fissure to the fissure of Sylvius.

(From Penfield and Rasmussen (1950) *The Cerebral Cortex of Man: a clinical study of localization of function.* Macmillan.)

position and cutaneous sensation terminate along the Rolandic fissure in areas representing the many body-parts from the leg at the top of the postcentral gyrus to the head, face and tongue at the bottom. These somato-sensory receiving areas are strikingly illustrated in Penfield's diagram, reproduced in Fig. 5, in which their relative sizes and positions are represented by the appropriate body areas of a homunculus.

As noted above these receiving areas in the cortex are quite small, but each is close to, or surrounded by, its primary association area to which it is connected by many association fibres. The auditory receiving area is connected (in animals) to the motor neurones which prick up the ear, the visual receiving area to the motor neurones of muscles directing the eye towards the source of the stimulus, and the post-Rolandic body areas to the motor neurones across the fissure which innervate the appropriate body muscles. A homunculus representing the motor areas lying along the precentral gyrus of the human cortex has also been designed by Penfield and is reproduced in Fig. 6.

The primary receiving areas are, however, not the only end-stations of afferent pathways to the cortex. Hearing, vision, and touch are each doubly, and possibly trebly, represented in each hemisphere with separate projection pathways, the pattern of representation being reversed in these subsidiary areas. The location of these secondary areas has been worked out in detail in animals, also in man, by stimulation during operations on the brain. The motor areas have also been found to have duplicates.

Until the mid-twentieth century it was customary to regard these specific afferent pathways for each sensory modality as the only route to the cortex for impulses coming from the periphery, but with the realisation of a non-specific system ascending in the mesial brain stem has come the recognition of a more intricate relationship of the brain with the environment. This development has resulted in an entirely new concept of brain mechanisms, and is the result of discoveries by Magoun and Moruzzi in the bulbar portion of the brain stem and of Morison and Dempsey in the diencephalon. These findings, essentially electrophysiological in nature, are discussed in greater detail in Chapter 17.

Some more diffuse association areas of the cortex are less directly connected to the receiving areas and are part of the general intercommunication system of the brain, a system entailing a hundred times as many neurones within the cortical layers as ever leave it. It has been calculated that the networks of neurones in the felt-work of the cortex are so numerous that an impulse entering by any single fibre could be routed directly or indirectly to every other neurone, but some process exists by which one abstracts from this mass of messages those of import at the time. This is well illustrated by Gerard's story of the small boy who, called on to read aloud in class, was asked the

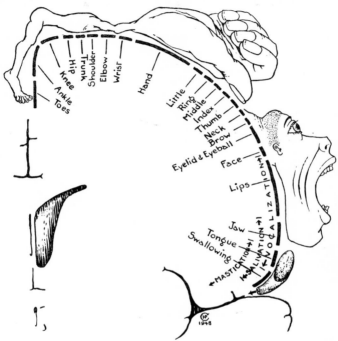

FIG. 6. MOTOR REPRESENTATION OF THE BODY IN THE PRECENTRAL
GYRUS

This is a motor homunculus designed by Penfield to show the motor representation of the various parts of the body in the precentral gyrus. (From Penfield and Rasmussen (1950) *The Cerebral Cortex of Man: a clinical study of localization of function.* Macmillan.)

meaning of what he had read and give the startled reply, 'I don't know. I wasn't listening.'

The spinal cord also consists of cell bodies and fibre tracts. The motor neurones, whose axons emerge from the cord through the ventral roots to innervate the voluntary muscles, have large cell bodies situated in the anterior grey matter of the spinal column. Some of these peripheral axons may be of great length; those of the sciatic nerve in man, for example, may reach a length of 3 feet or more. The cell bodies of the sensory neurones lie in the dorsal ganglia outside the cord and their

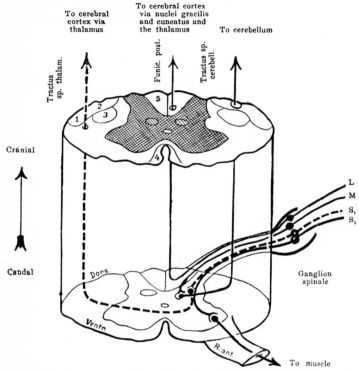

FIG. 7. SECTION OF SPINAL CORD TO ILLUSTRATE THE ENTRY OF AFFERENT FIBRES THROUGH THE DORSAL ROOT

Sympathetic efferents, descending branches and short interneurones (some of which cross to the opposite side) are not represented in this simplified diagram.

(From Bing and Haymaker (1956) *Regional Diagnosis of the Brain and Spinal Cord*. Mosby, St Louis.)

axons enter by the dorsal roots (Fig. 7). Lying wholly within the cord are interneurones of varying length.

Another division of the nervous system, the autonomic system, is responsible for the innervation of smooth muscle, of cardiac muscle, of the capillaries, and of the glands. It forms the efferent system to the viscera, whose afferent supply is through the sensory visceral nerves. Many of the cell bodies of the autonomic neurones are grouped in the ganglia of the vertebral chains lying alongside, and connecting with, the spinal cord. In the thoracic and lumbar segments this central connexion is made by the short myelinated fibres of the white rami, the system constituting the sympathetic division of the autonomic nervous system (Fig. 8). The efferent fibres from these ganglia

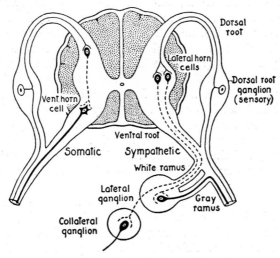

FIG. 8. THE CONNEXIONS OF AUTONOMIC FIBRES IN THE SPINAL CORD
(From Gaskell, redrawn in MacLeod (1956) *Physiology and Biochemistry in Modern Medicine*. Mosby, St Louis.)

are mostly unmyelinated and greatly exceed in number the preganglionic fibres, so that passage of impulses through a ganglion (where they meet their sole synapse) results in a widely-diffuse excitation. The other autonomic division, the parasympathetic, has its outflow in the cranial and sacral regions where the preganglionic fibres pass out in the ventral roots. Its synapses lie in, or close to, the organs it supplies, so that excitation in this system is more discretely localised. In general these two types of autonomic nerve have antagonistic actions on their effector organs.

The observation by Elliott that adrenaline mimics the effect of sympathetic activity, and the demonstration by Dale that acetylcholine may mimic parasympathetic action, are the fundamental discoveries in this field that have led to the formulation of a theory of chemical mediation of transmission in sympathetic and parasympathetic nerves. To use Cannon's generalisation, the prime function of the sympathetic division of the autonomic system is to maintain homeostasis of the internal environment, the 'milieu intérieur' of Claude Bernard, in spite of external stress, whereas that of the parasympathetic is to protect, conserve and restore the resources of the organism.

Wherever there is intercommunication between one cell and another the ultimate connexion between the two neurones is apparently across a gap, since in vertebrates there is no known continuity of nervous tissue from one cell to another. This gap is called the synapse, a word first used by Sherrington. The fine terminal branches of an axon may make connexion with other neurones through synapses onto cell bodies, onto dendrites or onto other axons. Since each axon may branch into many fibrils, and since each nerve cell has many dendrites, any single neurone may make interconnexions with a great many others.

The function of this immense network of interconnecting neurones which is the basic structure of the brain, cord and peripheral nerves, is to convey information from one part of the body to another. After hundreds of years of conjecturing about the nerve impulse, physiologists are still arguing about it, although they no longer 'anxiously discuss whether the spirit is carried along certain hollow channels of the nerves, or whether it passes through the solid material of the nerves.'

A great step forward was made when Du Bois-Reymond working in Berlin showed, in 1845, that a nervous impulse is always accompanied by the passage along the nerve of a change of electrical state. It is the nature of this electrical effect that is the subject of this book.

BIBLIOGRAPHY

Bard, P. (1937) Studies on the cortical representation of somatic sensibility. *Harvey Lect.*, **33**, 143–169.
Bing, R. and Haymaker, W. (1956) *Regional Diagnosis in Lesions of the Brain and Spinal Cord.* Mosby, St Louis.

Brief Outline of Physiology of the Nervous System   13

Bucy, P. D. (1949) *The Precentral Cortex*. University of Illinois Press.
Cannon, W. B. and Rosenblueth, A. (1937) *Autonomic Neuro-Effector Systems*. Macmillan, New York.
Dale, H. H. (1937) Transmission of nervous effects by acetylcholine. *Harvey Lect.*, **32**, 229–244.
Davson, H. (1964) *A Textbook of General Physiology*, 3rd ed. Little, Brown, Boston.
Elliot, T. R. (1904) On the action of adrenaline. *J. Physiol. (Lond.)*, **31**, 20–21.
Field, J., Magoun, H. W. and Hall, V. (Eds.) (1959, 1960) *Handbook of Physiology—Neurophysiology*. 3 vols. American Physiological Society, Washington.
Fulton, J. F. (1949) *Physiology of the Nervous System*, 3rd ed. Oxford University Press, London.
Lorente de Nó, R. (1947) *A Study of Nerve Physiology*. Rockefeller Institute, New York.
Lux, H. D. and Pollen, D. A. (1966) Electrical constants of neurons in the motor cortex of the cat. *J. Physiol. (Lond.)*, **29**, 207–220.
Macleod's *Physiology and Biochemistry in Modern Medicine*. Mosby, St Louis, 1956.
Magoun, H. W. (1950) Caudal and cephalic influences of the brain stem reticular formation. *Physiol. Rev.*, **30**, 459–474.
Moruzzi, G. (1950) *Problems in Cerebellar Physiology*. C. C. Thomas, Springfield.
Papez, J. W. (1948) *Human Growth and Development*. Cornell Co-operative Society.
Penfield, W. and Rasmussen, T. (1950) *The Cerebral Cortex of Man. A clinical study of localization of function*. Macmillan, New York.
Ramón y Cajal, S. (1952) *Histologie du Système Nerveux de l'Homme et des Vertébrés*. Maloine, Paris.
Ranson, S. W. and Clark, S. L. (1959) *The Anatomy of the Nervous System*. Saunders, Phila.
Rasmussen, A. T. (1932) *The Principal Nervous Pathways*. Macmillan, New York.
Ruch, T. C. and Patton, H. D. (1965) *Physiology and Biophysics*, 19th edition of Fulton and Howell's *Textbook of Physiology*. Saunders, Phila.
Sherrington, C. S. (1947) *The Integrative Action of the Nervous System*, 2nd ed. Cambridge University Press, Cambridge.
Wright, S. (1965) *Applied Physiology*, 11th ed. Oxford University Press, London.

2

The Electrical Change Associated with Nervous Activity in Axons

THE nerve impulse is not an electric current flowing down the length of the fibre in the way that electricity passes down a wire, but is a progression of ionic changes whose electrical signs constitute the action potential. The energy for the transmission of the impulse comes from the nerve itself and not from the stimulus. As the wave of activity travels along the neurone, each point it reaches becomes electrically negative to the inactive regions on each side of it. As the impulse passes down the nerve the length of the travelling region of activity which shows a potential change from the resting state is called the wave-length. In very fine fibres this measures only a few millimetres or so, but in large A fibres the wave-length may be as much as 5 or even 6 cm. Thus, if one places two recording electrodes on an isolated nerve suspended in air, or in any other non-conducting medium, as in Fig. 9, any adequate recording system will register a sudden negative potential on the external surface of the fibre as the wave of activity passes the first electrode (a) since this is now negative to the second electrode (b). As the wave of activity proceeds to electrode (b) this will now in its turn become negative to the first, and the current flow will be reversed through the instrument. The apparent reversal of polarity is due to the electrodes being connected to opposite inputs of the recording instrument.

The record one obtains is, therefore, that of the upward deflection* of the negative potential change at the first electrode, followed by a downward deflection as the second electrode

* It is common usage among electrophysiologists to connect the input terminals of their recording instruments in such a way that when the electrode over active tissue becomes relatively negative to an electrode over inactive tissue, an upward deflection is produced in their records. This is, of course, an arbitrary convention, and is opposite to that most commonly used in the physical sciences.

becomes negative to the first, in other words, a wave followed by its inverted mirror image. The interval between the negative phase and the positive is determined by the time it takes for the impulse to travel from the first electrode to the second,

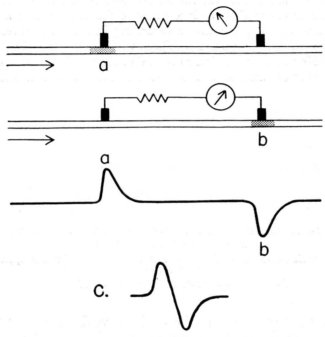

FIG. 9. THE PASSAGE OF A NERVE IMPULSE IN A NON-CONDUCTING MEDIUM

The resultant recording is obtained as the wave of activity passes consecutively under two electrodes both of which are on the nerve. The record obtained when the two electrodes are close together, as shown at c, gives the appearance of a diphasic wave. It should be noted that in the upper two diagrams the abscissa represents length in space, and in the lower two it represents passage of time.

that is, on the distance between them and on the conduction velocity of the nerve. If the electrodes are very close together the two parts of the doubly-recorded wave become partially superimposed.

The potential changes under the first electrode are the electrical sign of the nerve impulse at a single region in the nerve, and the record of them is universally known as the action potential of nerve. By the simple expedient of crushing or otherwise damaging the area under the second electrode the effects of the passage of the impulse under the first electrode can be studied alone without the subsequent results of its passing the second electrode. Such a study of the monophasic action potential with more sensitive recording instruments reveals it to have several components. These will be described in detail later. Nervous conduction never takes place without this electrical change and it has the same essential characteristics

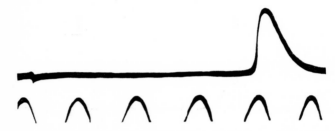

FIG. 10. MONOPHASIC SPIKE POTENTIAL OF SINGLE UNMYELINATED AXON OF CRAB NERVE IN OIL

The small deflection on the left signals when the stimulus was applied. Time in msec.

(From Hodgkin (1939) *J. Physiol.* (*Lond.*), **94**, 560.)

whether one records from the single nerve fibre or the nerve trunk, from the sensory nerve or from the motor nerve. A classical monophasic action potential in a single nerve fibre is shown in Fig. 10.

The wave of activity produces not only an electrical effect as it passes, but also a small amount of heat. Each of these effects is very small. The potential difference across the membrane is only about a tenth of a volt lasting for a few thousandths of a second, and a single impulse raises the temperature only one four-millionth of a degree centigrade, but the speed with which the impulse travels is very fast (about 200 miles an hour in some nerves in man), the exact speed depending on the size of the fibre involved.

The physico-chemical processes behind the production of the potential changes are still not established beyond dispute, but there is little doubt that there is only one kind of nerve impulse and that this is universal to the nervous system. The conduction of this nerve impulse is the principal function of the nerve fibres.

The metabolism of resting nerve is an oxidative one demanding oxygen and substrate and producing carbon dioxide and a small quantity of heat. The principal substrate is glucose which, together with phospholipids, supplies the energy necessary to maintain the resting state. Evidence is, however, lacking that either of these is the source of the energy for the conduction of the nerve impulse which is only indirectly dependent on oxygen supply. The passage of the nerve impulse takes energy from the fibre for its propagation and this is thought to come not from glucose but from the breakdown of phosphocreatine which contains energy-rich phosphate bonds. The role of acetylcholine in nerve metabolism was the subject of a controversy which is outlined in a later chapter.

The chemical reactions involved are on such a small scale that their detection has necessitated very careful and intricate methods of measurement. From a series of studies extending over a long period Hill was able to establish that the passage of a nerve impulse is accompanied by a heat production of approximately 10^{-7} small calories per gramme of nerve fibre. The major part of the heat produced is clearly related to the restorative process since it is maximal during the recovery period. Only a small fraction of heat is given off during the initial phase of the action potential and Hill interpreted this as due to the partial discharge of an electrical double layer located at the surface of the fibre. Active nerve consumes about a third as much again of oxygen as does the resting nerve, but most of this is absorbed not during the action spike but in the recovery period during the phase of maximal heat production in the process of restoring the resting condition. There is a corresponding rise in carbon dioxide output.

A detailed discussion of the chemical processes in nerve is outside the scope of this book. In brief it may be noted that the maintenance of the resting potential and its restoration after the passage of a nerve impulse seem to be oxidative processes involving glucose metabolism, whereas a different reaction is responsible for the energy for nerve conduction. A discussion of the roles of potassium and of sodium will be found in the section on the propagation of the nerve impulse.

The importance of nerve impulses lies, not in their energy characteristics, but in their role as signals in a communication system for establishing a degree of order that can lead to effectiveness of function.

BIBLIOGRAPHY

Abbott, B. C. (1960) Heat production in nerve and electric organ. *J. gen. Physiol.*, **43**, Suppl., 119–127.

Abood, L. G. (1960) Neuronal metabolism. In *Handbook of Physiology, Neurophysiology*. Amer. Physiol. Soc. Washington, Vol. 3, 1815–1826.

Adrian, E. D. (1914) The all-or-none principle in nerve. *J. Physiol.*, **47**, 460–474.

Adrian, E. D. (1932) *The Mechanism of Nervous Action*. Pennsylvania Press.

Brink, F., Bronk, D. W., Carlson, F. D. and Connelly, C. M. (1952) The oxygen uptake of active axons. *Cold Spr. Har. Symp. Quant. Biol.*, **17**, 53–67.

Gasser, H. S. (1941) The classification of nerve fibres. *Ohio J. Sci.*, **41**, 145–159.

Gerard, R. W. (1932) Nerve metabolism. *Physiol. Rev.*, **12**, 469–592.

Hill, A. V. (1932) *Chemical Wave Transmission in Nerve*. Cambridge University Press.

Hill, A. V. (1960) The heat production of nerve. In *Molecular Biology*. Academic Press, New York, 153–162.

Hodgkin, A. L. (1964) *The Conduction of the Nervous Impulse*. Thomas, Springfield, 108 pp.

Hydén, H. (1960) The neuron. In *The Cell: Biochemistry, Physiology, Morphology*. Academic Press, New York, 215–323.

Keynes, R. D. (1960) The effect of complete and partial inhibition of metabolism on active transport in nerve and muscle. In *Regulation of the Inorganic Ion Content of Cells*. Little, Brown, Boston, 77–88.

McIlwain, H. (1959) *Biochemistry and the Central Nervous System*. Little, Brown, Boston, 2nd edition.

McIlwain, H. (1963) *Chemical Exploration of the Brain*. Elsevier, Amsterdam.

3
Action Potentials in Peripheral Nerve Recorded By External Electrodes

RECORDING the action potential from nerves in man has obvious difficulties. Most of our detailed knowledge has therefore been derived from the nerves of animals.

When a stimulus of any kind (mechanical, thermal, chemical, or electrical) is applied to a nerve, the nerve being irritable, reacts. This property of irritability is the most important characteristic of nerve, and knowledge of its mechanism has advanced immeasurably with the technique originally developed by Adrian and Bronk for studying isolated nerve fibres. However, a great deal of the ground-work was established by study of the classical muscle-nerve preparation consisting of a single muscle with its supplying nerve trunk. Each development in recording technique has made its contribution to electrophysiology and this is especially true of thermionic valve amplification. Recording instruments have evolved through the capillary electrometer, the Einthoven string galvanometer, and electromagnetic recorders, to the cathode-ray oscilloscope. The last-named device with its inertia-less electron beam has proved to be the instrument of choice for the recording of the exceedingly brief and feeble currents of nerve.

One of the basic conditions of nervous conduction is the 'all-or-nothing' principle. This important law states that, provided an impulse is strong enough to be propagated, the size of the response, and the speed of its conduction will be independent of the intensity of the stimulus. The response is all that the nerve can give at the moment and nothing less. Bowditch discovered this type of effect in 1871 when working with heart muscle, but the work of Lucas and Adrian showed that this principle applies not only to muscle but to the axons of nerves.

The all-or-nothing law was thought for years to apply to all electrical activity in neurones—to the nerve cell itself, to the receptor and effector endings, and to the dendrites. Happily for those who strive to find the mechanisms that code the subtle reactions of the nervous system, it is now known that in the mammalian nervous system this restrictive behaviour is confined only to the propagated discharge, and many finer electrical changes of a graded sort have been detected and defined at both the peripheral and central ends of these conducting fibres as well as in the receptor organs, thus providing greater plasticity of reaction. The all-or-nothing principle still stands, however, for the propagated discharge in the conducting portion of the neurone.

It follows that the state of the fibre at the point where the stimulus is applied becomes all-important in deciding the size of the response. Should the fibre be exhausted by the very recent passage of an impulse, or by inadequate oxygen supply, or be narcotised by some drug, then the size of response may be reduced. This is not surprising when one remembers that the energy for the transmission of the impulse comes from metabolic processes within the nerve itself and not from the stimulus.

Taking the first of these situations, that of the fibre along which an impulse has just passed: each response is followed by a period of refractoriness which follows the impulse down the whole length of the nerve during which no stimulus however strong can be effective. Forbes described this as the 'line-busy' effect. For a fraction of a second the nerve fibre is incapable of transmitting another impulse. Following this state of absolute refractoriness is a period of relative refractoriness when the membrane of the nerve fibre is in the process of recovering from depolarisation, so that only a stimulus of more than the usual strength is able to excite it, but provided this new threshold is attained, the response will be all-or-nothing.

Similarly if the nerve is impaired by a narcotic its excitability will be reduced. In the case where a section only of the nerve is thus impaired, the response from this section only will be subnormal, areas of nerve on either side of it giving the full responses.

Within limits, where the nerve has a normal energy supply available, the transmission will be normal and where it is locally impaired the response will also be locally impaired. The size of the impulse at a given place in the nerve is determined only by the state of the fibre at that place and is not affected by its having just traversed sections of impaired nerve. This was clearly demonstrated by Davis and Forbes and their colleagues in their experiments on nerves in a narcotising chamber. They found reduction of response from the section of nerve within the chamber but no progressive decrement along its narcotised length and no accumulative effect of impairment; the section of nerve emerging from the narcotising chamber gave full responses. Kato's pioneer work had given similar results, and the old hypothesis of 'decremental conduction' was proved no longer tenable.

Since, in the unimpaired nerve, the size of the conducted response is independent of the intensity of stimulus, some other characteristics must be responsible for differentiating between weak and strong stimuli. In the nerve trunk the number of fibres stimulated increases with the size of the stimulus, but in the single fibre the only gradation with intensity is in the frequency of recurrent impulses in the fibre. A single impulse may cause a muscle-unit twitch, but a stream of impulses following each other down the many fibres of a nerve can hold a muscle in contraction; the higher the frequency the greater the contraction. It is usually said that in man the frequency of nerve impulses per fibre which maintains a muscle, such as the biceps, in steady contraction has been calculated to be about 50/sec, and for tone in maintaining the erect posture, about 10/sec. It is more likely, however, that recruitment of extra fibres is the more important factor in intense voluntary contraction.

Another property of nerve which is independent of the strength of the stimulus is the velocity at which the nerve impulse is conducted along the fibre. In any given fibre the impulse set up by a strong stimulus travels no faster than that from a weak stimulus (although the rate differs in different types of fibre).

The measurement of conduction velocity in nerve has been the subject of study ever since the experiments of Helmholtz in 1850. He invented a 'myograph' by which he measured for the first time the velocity of the nerve impulse. Since then many observations have followed, mostly based on measurements of motor or sensory reaction times, but a clear understanding only became possible with the recognition by Erlanger and Gasser, and by Bishop and Heinbecker, of the different types of fibre of which nerves are composed. The three types of fibre have been given no names other than the first three letters of the alphabet; the A fibres are the largest (the myelinated fibres of somatic nerves), the B fibres are the small thinly-myelinated fibres (the fibres of visceral nerves), and the C group, which are the smallest, have little apparent myelin. A fibres are found in both motor and sensory nerves, B in autonomic ones and C fibres in sympathetic nerves and in dorsal spinal roots. The two sub-categories of C fibres have somewhat different characteristics in their action potential sequences.

A nerve impulse travels fastest in an A fibre, less fast in a B fibre, and slowest in a C fibre; and in the mammalian A fibres themselves the velocity at which the nerve impulse travels bears a relationship to the diameter of the axon: the thicker the axon the faster the conduction.

Gasser and Erlanger from their studies concluded at first that the velocity varied as the square of the diameter, and then from later experiments that the relationship of velocity to diameter was a linear one. The accumulated evidence from many sources would point to the relationship being directly proportional to the diameter of invertebrate and myelinated mammalian nerve (including the myelin), and proportional to the square root of the diameter in the unmyelinated nerves of vertebrates.

Where an axon arborises into terminal branches, these branches conduct at a reduced velocity. For example, Holmgren has found a reduction from 20 m/sec to 2 m/sec in the dorsal tracts of the frog's spinal cord as the fibres branch or give off collaterals.

In man these myelinated A fibres vary from 1/1000th to 1/50th of a millimetre in diameter, which, if the same factor relationship holds for man as for animals, would indicate conduction velocities varying from about 8 to 140 m/sec. This type of fibre carries impulses set up by touch, by pressure and by position sense in the muscles as well as being the archetype of the motor nerve fibre.

Pain fibres in man conduct more slowly (from 4 to 20 m/sec) but the type of fibre conveying painful sensation is still a matter for debate—the conduction velocity is often too fast for C fibres and it may possibly be that small myelinated A fibres are also involved.

In the sympathetic nervous system in man the conduction velocity is slower again (about 2 m/sec) in the postganglionic fibres. These are apparently unmyelinated fibres mostly of the C type and, therefore, the slowest to conduct, though they differ in some respects from the C fibres in the dorsal roots. It should, however, be recognised that there is evidence from the latest work on the ultrastructure of nerve that even these fibres may in fact carry a thin coat of myelin. There is also a relationship between the excitability of a fibre and its conduction velocity— the faster a nerve conducts the greater its excitability.

ACTION POTENTIAL IN SINGLE 'A' FIBRES OF PERIPHERAL NERVE

Much of our detailed knowledge of the action potential of peripheral nerve we owe to Gasser and Erlanger and to their colleagues and pupils, but the technique by which it may be studied in the single fibre we owe to Adrian and Bronk. Of necessity the first work was done on animals, but great constancy in electrical characteristics has been found among mammals, and modern techniques show that man is no exception.

The fastest conducting fibres in mammalian nerves are the A type which vary in diameter from 20μ to 1μ. In these fibres the action potential is always made up of the same three components: the spike, the negative after-potential, and the positive after-potential.

These properties when first discovered were described phenomenologically but, since the developments of techniques for penetrating the axon and recording directly from inside, the more intimate transmembrane potential changes underlying the genesis of the spike potential and the negative and positive after-potentials have now been studied (as described later in this book).

The Spike Potential in Peripheral Axons. The spike is by far the greatest in magnitude of the three components, and has the shortest duration (about 1/2 msec in mammalian A fibres). Its magnitude does not change however strong the stimulus and does not fall off however long the fibre along which it is propagated. In other words it acts according to the all-or-nothing principle. The size of the spike recorded externally to the axon depends only on the type of fibre and on the state of that fibre when it receives the stimulus; since the amplitude of the spike varies with the diameter of the fibre it also varies with its conduction velocity. Thus, an A-type fibre of large diameter and rapid conduction will give a larger spike potential than a smaller fibre. At constant temperature, the duration of the spike is constant in all mammalian A fibres, the rising phase of the potential taking up about one-third of the total time, and the falling phase two-thirds at body temperature. The spike, with

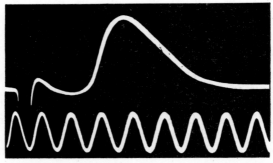

FIG. II. MONOPHASIC SPIKE POTENTIAL IN A SINGLE A FIBRE OF A
CAT'S NERVE IN OIL, RECORDED EXTERNALLY

Distance between recording electrodes: 1 cm. Temperature 32°C. The break in the record on the left signals the moment of stimulation. Time signal: 5,000 c/s.
(From Rosenblueth, Wiener, Pitts and Ramos (1948) *J. cell. comp. Physiol.*, **32**, 275.)

its extremely stable characteristics, is the basic unit of the action potential and is that part of it which is associated with the passage of the nerve impulse. During the passage of a single nerve impulse in an A fibre about 5 cm of nerve is active at any one moment (less in smaller fibres).

An accurate illustration of the spike potential, taken from Rosenblueth, is shown in Fig. II. Unlike some of the representations of action spikes that have been published, this shows minimal distortion by the amplifying system, one of the major errors which mars many other records of the spike. The shape of the spike shown here, established by Rosenblueth on A fibres of mammalian myelinated nerve, has been found to be identical with that recorded by Hodgkin from unmyelinated crustacean nerve, as can be seen by comparing Fig. 11 with Fig. 10. Rosenblueth and Wiener have computed the mathematical equations for this curve and from these calculations infer that three consecutive physiological events contribute to the action spike. The nature of these events will become clearer in Chapters 6 and 8.

The velocity of the nerve impulse is highest in mammalian A fibres where it reaches about 100–120 m/sec at body temperature, or less than one-third of the speed of sound. In cold-blooded animals it is slower (about 30 m/sec in the frog at

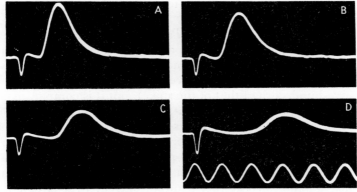

FIG. 12. THE EFFECT OF TEMPERATURE ON THE MONOPHASIC SPIKE
POTENTIAL IN A SINGLE FIBRE OF CAT'S NERVE RECORDED
EXTERNALLY

Temperatures: *A*, 37·7°C; *B*, 33·0°C; *C*, 27·2°C; *D*, 24·0°C. The downward deflection on the left of each record signals the moment of stimulation. Time signal: 2,000 c/s.

(From Rosenblueth, Wiener, Pitts and Ramos (1948) *J. cell. comp. Physiol.*, **32**, 275.)

20°C) but in all species which have both types of nerve it is faster in myelinated than in unmyelinated nerve. It is greatly influenced by a change in temperature, as also are the amplitude of the spike (which decreases with decreasing temperature) and the duration of the spike (which increases). An illustration of this effect is seen in Fig. 12.

The Negative After-potential in Peripheral Axons Recorded Externally. This phase begins before the spike has returned to zero potential; it represents a residual depolarisation and its beginning is seen as a break in the smooth decline of the spike potential, decreasing the speed of fall. In mammalian A fibres the greatest size which this potential reaches is only about one-twentieth of that of the spike, but it lasts much longer—15 msec. It lasts longer still after rapidly repeated stimulation (i.e. tetanus), increasing in duration with the frequency of the stimuli.

Unlike the spike the negative after-potential is very variable and is easily affected by metabolic and environmental conditions, including levels of anoxia or acidity which may not affect the spike. Even when the asphyxia is intense enough completely to abolish the after-potentials the spike will persist.

The Positive After-potential in Peripheral Axons Recorded Externally. When the negative after-potential has ended, the potential does not remain at the baseline value but falls to the positive side. This positive phase is of very low potential (only about one-five-hundredth of that of the spike), but it is comparatively long-lasting, persisting for about 70 msec or longer. Like the negative after-potential it is responsive to changes in metabolism or environment, but is more constant in its time-relations to the spike. The positive after-potential at the end of a long tetanus is indistinguishable from the effect of the 'make' of an applied anodal current (i.e. a direct current in a circuit the anode of which lies on the nerve and the cathode on some remote inactive tissue). After-potentials reflect changes in membrane conductance following the spike. The negative after-potential is a slow repolarisation which is then succeeded by a long-lasting phase of hyperpolarisation.

A glance at the relative magnitude and time-durations of the three components of the action potential makes immediately apparent the difficulty of studying simultaneously the full sequence of potential changes. The instrument of choice is the cathode-ray oscilloscope, since the deflection of the electron beam can respond without delay to the rapidly-changing potential of the spike potential and the time base can be made logarithmic on the screen, but amplification for magnitude of the components remains a problem. The various components are, therefore, usually studied separately. The same difficulties accompany the depicting of the results of such study. A time scale is needed which is fast enough to reveal the duration of the

upward rise of the spike deflection (0·12 msec), yet projecting
far enough to include the end of the positive after-potential
100 msec later. A logarithmic time-scale still leaves the difficulty of depicting clearly the deviation from zero of the positive
after-potential which at its maximum is only 0·2 per cent of
that of the spike. Consequently a convention has arisen by
which the full magnitude of the spike is not reproduced but is

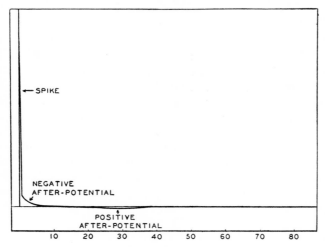

FIG. 13. DIAGRAMMATIC RECONSTRUCTION OF THE ACTION
POTENTIAL

This demonstrates the relative sizes of the spike and after-potentials and
their time-relationships in *A* fibres. Time in msec.
(Redrawn from Gasser (1937) *Harvey Lect.*, **32** 169.)

indicated in the legend accompanying the chart. Fig. 13, redrawn from Gasser's original diagram, is a reconstruction of
the action potential sequence in an A fibre. The scale necessary
to include the whole of the spike makes the positive after-
potential almost invisible. This is the reason why the after-
potentials are not visible in Figs. 10, 11 and 12.

When the properties of each component of the nerve action
potential are studied in this way the role which each plays in
assuring that the parts of the body have a delicately-adjustable
system of intercommunication becomes clearer. The spike
potential is the steady reliable concomitant of the passage of

the nerve impulse following faithfully the all-or-nothing principle, whereas the after-potentials reflect the state of preparedness of the fibre to receive the stimulus, or, as Gasser has put it, 'If the spikes may be called the message carriers of the nervous system, the after-potentials in contrast may be called the indicators of the readiness with which messages will be accepted.'

ACTION POTENTIALS IN SINGLE 'B' FIBRES OF
    PERIPHERAL NERVE

Mammalian B fibres were first studied extensively by Grundfest in the cat and by Bishop and Heinbecker in the rabbit. Their diameter is usually less than 3μ and their action potential differs from that of mammalian A fibres in that there is no apparent negative after-potential. Although there is no negative after-potential visible under ordinary conditions one can be brought out by special procedures such as repetitive stimuli. The positive after-potential is, however, very prominent in B fibres, being almost one-tenth of the magnitude of the spike, and it may last as long as one-third of a second. The spike is of longer duration than in the A fibre (1·2 msec) and, the fibre being of smaller diameter, the conduction velocity is less, never being more than 15 m/sec.

ACTION POTENTIALS IN 'C' FIBRES OF PERIPHERAL
    NERVE

At present few records of the action potential of single C fibres have yet been made owing to the difficulty of stimulating a fibre with such high threshold and slow conduction (less than 2 msec) without masking the response by the stimulus artefact, but in sympathetic nerve trunks whose composition is almost entirely of C fibres it is evident that there are both negative and positive after-potentials, in fact yet another negative after-potential seems to follow the positive one. In such nerves containing several C fibres the spike potential is found to last about 2 msec, and the negative after-potential 50–80 msec (see Fig. 14). The positive after-potential of sympathetic C fibres is the longest-lasting of the whole range of electrical responses set up by a single shock to a nerve: it is still traceable 2 seconds after the initial stimulus. The after-potentials of C fibres are much more resistant to changes in their environment, such as anoxia or acidity than are those of A and B fibres. In contrast to the C fibres of the autonomic system, those which are axons of cells in the dorsal-root ganglia of the spinal cord show no after-potentials of the kind described here. They exhibit an immediate post-spike reversal of sign to a positivity that may be in size as much as 30 per cent of the initial negative spike height.

When a comparison is made of the properties of the action potential in A, B and C fibres respectively it will be noted that

FIG. 14. ACTION SPIKE OF C FIBRES; SPLENIC NERVE OF THE CAT
Note the long duration of the spike compared with that of *A* fibres, and the long-lasting positive after-potential. Time signal: 60 c/s.
(From Gasser (1937) *Harvey Lect.*, **32**, 169.)

these differ quantitatively, both in magnitude and duration, although all contain essentially the same components. In the following table, adapted from Grundfest, the characteristics which have been described are summarised and the relationships between such properties as the size of fibre, conduction velocity, duration of refractory period, can be readily seen.

One of the many properties of the after-potentials of nerves is their tendency to swing into oscillation with changing ionic environment. An increase in the pH of the medium or an immobilisation of the Ca ion by addition of citrate is effective in bringing out a marked oscillation of excitability of the nerve. This is of especial interest in connexion with the inherent rhythmicity of nerve cells and will be referred to again.

One of the most important fundamentals of nerve electrophysiology is the fact that the component parts of the individual neurone have different electrical properties, just as they have different anatomical structure (dendrites, cell body, unmyelinated section of axon, and axon). But the variations in electrical characteristics are even greater in number than these morphological divisions, for some zones of the cell membrane, for

TABLE I

Properties of Three Groups of Mammalian Nerve Fibres
(adapted from Grundfest and from Gasser)

Group	A	B	C sympathetic	C dorsal root
Diameters of fibres in microns	20 to 1	< 3		1·2 = 0·4
Conduction velocity in m/sec	100 to < 5	14 to < 3	< 2	< 2·4
Spike duration in msec	0·4 to 0·5	1·2	2·0	2·0
Negative after-potential: *Amount* per cent of spike / *Duration* in msec	3 to 5 / 12 to 20	None / —	3 to 5 / 50 to 80	None / —
Positive after-potential: *Amount* per cent of spike / *Duration* in msec	0·2 / 40 to 60	1·5 to 4·0 / 100 to 300	1·5 / 300 to < 1000	Early reversal
Absolutely refractory period in msec	0·4α 0·6δ, cat 1·0δ, rabbit	1·2	2·0	— —
Period of latent addition in msec	0·2	0·2	2·5	—
Order of susceptibility to asphyxia	2	1	3	—

example, may have different properties from others, even from neighbouring zones. That this must be so was argued *a priori* before the development of microelectrode techniques. Before recordings could be made directly from within the cell, only changing potential, i.e. current flow, could be detected. Were all parts of the neurone to have identical properties (identical discharge time, recovery time, degree of polarisation, etc.) no current would flow outside the neurone itself and hence no external potential changes could occur to be recorded by extra-cellular electrodes.

But, in fact, the electrical properties of the various parts of a neurone are so different that a change in polarisation level at any one point causes current to flow between that point and other parts of the neurone. The potential changes due to these current flows are what have been categorised as pre-potentials, spike potentials and after-potentials.

An example of the physical property of membrane that may vary from one part of the neurone to another is its time-constant. This term is used in neurophysiology in the same sense as its original use in the theory of electrical networks. When a rectangular current pulse is applied to the nerve the potential across the membrane does not rise to maximum immediately but increases gradually with an exponential curve. The time constant is defined (as for electrical networks) as the time taken for this curve to approach $1/e$ of the final value and this depends entirely on the product of the resistance and capacitance of the membrane. Were there no capacitance the time constant would be zero. Motor neurones have been found to have a time constant of approximately 2·5 msec.

The evolution of electrodes small enough to penetrate the neurone itself has made possible the direct measurement of potential difference across the membrane in the absence of current flow. In the large cells of the motor neurones of the spinal cord this standing potential difference has been measured to be 70 μV (inside negative to outside of the membrane). This, of course, is a measurement of the potential averaged over the cell and gives no information about zones within the cell that may differ from each other in potential.

The time taken to recover from a propagated spike is one of the outstanding differences between the cell body of the motor neurone and its axon—the absolute refractory period lasts only $\frac{1}{2}$ msec for the axon but is from 2 to 2·5 msec long for the cell body. The period of subnormality is as long as 100 to 150 msec for the cell, and considerably shorter for the axon. These dis-similarities result in extracellular current flows that can be detected by electrodes lying outside the neurone.

BIBLIOGRAPHY

Adrian, E. D. (1912) On the conduction of subnormal disturbances in normal nerve. *J. Physiol. (Lond.)*, **45**, 389–412.

Adrian, E. D. (1914) The all-or-none principle in nerve. *J. Physiol. (Lond.)*, **47**, 460–474.

Adrian, E. D. and Bronk, D. W. (1928) The discharge of impulses in motor nerve fibres. I. Impulses in single fibres of the phrenic nerve. *J. Physiol. (Lond.)*, **66**, 81–101.

Adrian, E. D. and Bronk, D. W. (1929) The discharge of impulses in motor nerve fibres. II. The frequency of discharge in reflex and voluntary contractions. *J. Physiol. (Lond.)*, **67**, 119–151.

Bishop, G. H. and Heinbecker, P. (1930) Differentiation of axon types in visceral nerves by means of the potential record. *Amer. J. Physiol.*, **94**, 170–200.

Bowditch, H. P. (1871) Über die Eigenthumlichkeiten der Reizbarkeit welche die Muskelfasern des Herzens zeigen. *Ber. Sachs. Ges. Wiss.*, **23**, 652–689.

Coombs, J. S., Eccles, J. C. and Fatt, P. (1955) The electrical properties of the motorneurone membrane. *J. Physiol. (Lond.)*, **130**, 291–325.

Davis, H., Forbes, A., Brunswick, D. and Hopkins, A. McH. (1926) Studies of nerve impulse: question of decrement. *Amer. J. Physiol.*, **76**, 448–471.

Erlanger, J. and Gasser, H. (1937) *Electrical Signs of Nervous Activity.* University of Pennsylvania Press.

Gasser, H. S. (1955) Properties of dorsal root unmedullated fibres on the two sides of the ganglion. *J. gen. Physiol.*, **38**, 709–728.

Gasser, H. and Grundfest, H. (1939) Axon diameters in relation to spike dimensions and conduction velocity in mammalian fibres. *Amer. J. Physiol.*, **127**, 393–414.

Grundfest, H. (1939) The properties of mammalian B. fibres. *Amer. J. Physiol.*, **127**, 252–262.

Grundfest, H. and Gasser, H. S. (1938) Properties of mammalian nerve fibres of slowest conduction. *Amer. J. Physiol.*, **123**, 307–318.

von Helmholtz, H. (1850) Messungen über die zeitlichen Verlauf der Zuckung animalischer Muskeln und die Fortpflanzungsgeschwindigkeit der Reizung in den Nerven. *Arch. Anat. Physiol.*, 277–364.

Hodes, R. (1953) Linear relationship between fibre diameter and velocity of conduction in giant axon of the squid. *J. Neurophysiol.*, **16**, 145–154.

Hodgkin, A. L. and Katz, B. (1949) The effect of temperature on the electrical activity of the giant axon of the squid. *J. Physiol. (Lond.)*, **109**, 240–249.

Holmgren, B. (1954) Conduction along dorsal tracts of spinal cord. *J. Physiol. (Lond.)*, **123**, 324–337.

Hursh, J. B. (1939) Conduction velocity and diameter of nerve fibres. *Amer. J. Physiol.*, **127**, 131–139.

Kato, G. (1924) *The Theory of Decrementless Conduction in Narcotised Region of Nerve.* Nankodo, Tokyo.

Kato, G. (1926) *Further Studies on Decrementless Conduction.* Nankodo, Tokyo.

Rosenblueth, A., Wiener, N., Pitts, W. and Garcia Ramos, J. (1948) An account of the spike potential of axons. *J. cell comp. Physiol.*, **32**, 275–317.

Rushton, W. A. H. (1951) A theory of the effects of fibre size in medullated nerve. *J. Physiol. (Lond.)*, **115**, 101–122.

4

The Excitability of Peripheral Nerve

WHAT is the underlying condition of the nerve while these complex changes of electrical potential are succeeding one another? Is it uniformly excitable all the time? These questions have been answered by studying the effect of introducing a second stimulus at the various stages of the action potential sequence. It is clear that there is a very close correlation between the potentials of a nerve fibre and its excitability, the three phases of potential change (the spike, the negative after-potential, and the positive after-potential) being accompanied by three distinct levels of excitability: the refractory period, the supernormal period, and the subnormal period. The specific meaning of the word 'excitability,' as it will be used here, is the reciprocal of the stimulation threshold.

In normal nerve the propagated impulse far exceeds in stimulating strength the threshold excitability of the fibre along which it is travelling; this excess (which may be as great as 10 : 1) is known as the factor of safety. In a nerve which has not had time to recover from the passage of a previous impulse this safety margin is wiped out by the rise in threshold known as the refractory period.

Most of the basic information about excitability of nerve and its periods of refractoriness was initially gathered from experiments on nerve trunks chosen for uniformity of fibre size. More modern techniques have extended this study to the behaviour of single nerve fibres, with essentially the same results.

The Refractory Period in Peripheral Axons. In 1889 Gotch and Burch using a capillary electrometer first showed that the second of two stimuli to a nerve will produce no response if it follows too closely on the first. The fibre needs about one one-thousandth of a second or more in which to recover from the passage of the first spike potential before it can transmit another. Closer study reveals that the refractory period itself has two parts, the first in which no stimulus, however strong, will excite the fibre (the absolutely refractory period) and the second when the nerve can be excited only if the stimulus is of more than normal threshold strength (the relatively refractory period).

The time relations of these excitability changes show the period of absolute refractoriness to coincide approximately with the rise of the spike potential and with its decline to the point where the negative after-potential distorts its falling curve. At this point the nerve again becomes excitable but has a high threshold, and so needs a more intense stimulus before it will respond. In other words, it is relatively refractory; this state is approximately coincident with the period of transition from the spike potential to the negative after-potential. The relationship between the duration of the spike potential and that of the absolutely refractory period is by no means exact. Although both are affected by temperature changes the refractory period shows a greater relative change at extremes of temperature.

During the absolutely refractory period the nerve is to all intents and purposes inert; not only is it impossible to evoke a second response anywhere along the nerve but it is also impossible to prolong the refractoriness by putting in a second stimulus during this period, although it has been demonstrated by Rosenblueth that this may augment the response to another stimulus falling in the relatively refractory period of the first. Hence, although unresponsive during the absolutely refractory period, the nerve is apparently not unchanged. Perhaps the word 'absolute' may be a misnomer for this phase.

As we have seen, the spike potential is the electrical signal of the nervous impulse, so we can now calculate the maximum number of impulses per second that can travel down a single fibre. In mammalian A fibres the period when the nerve is absolutely inexcitable being at body temperature about 0·5 msec, a stimulus, however strong, cannot evoke a response more often than 2,000 times in a second. This number, calculated arithmetically, has been confirmed experimentally. However, in natural conditions in the body the frequency of consecutive impulses in any fibre is more usually 10–100/sec and rarely reaches more than 500/sec. There is thus a large margin available to deal with an unusually intense stimulus. The refractory period is longer in the nerves of cold-blooded animals, as also is the duration of the action spike.

A new stimulus given at the beginning of the period of relative refractoriness will produce a smaller electrical response than normal and this will travel at a slower conduction rate than usual. This is illustrated in Fig. 15, in which several records from a frog are superimposed so that the response to the first shock is identically placed in every case. The earlier the second stimulus is introduced during the period of relative refractoriness, the smaller is the response from the nerve. Only when the

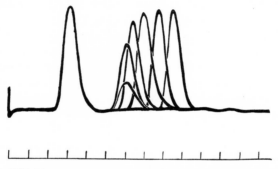

FIG. 15. THE RELATIVELY REFRACTORY PERIOD OF MOTOR FIBRES
IN FROG'S NERVE

Successive pictures have been superimposed so that the first responses are coincident. Paired maximal stimuli were given, the second following the first at intervals of 1·4, 1·6, 2·0, 2·6, 3·6 and 4·4 msec.
(From von Brücke, Early and Forbes (1941) *J. Neurophysiol.*, **4**, 80.)

interval approaches 4 msec is the second response fully sized in this cold-blooded animal. Again, clearly something has happened to the nerve as a result of the first stimulus which makes it unable to behave normally; some change has taken place from which the nerve has to recover before it can again give a full response, and this recovery process does not start until the original impulse is over. The spike is a sign of movement of negative ions outward through the membrane and of positive ions inward from the neighbouring inactive areas, but the nature of the physicochemical change involved in this ionic movement is not yet fully understood. As there has been more than one hypothesis advanced to explain it, this will be the subject of a separate chapter (Chapter 6), but whatever may be the nature of the process some facts are known; for example, this process needs a definite period for recovery; and we know something else about it: more heat is liberated during this re- covery phase than during the production of the spike. The energy for the spike potential and the energy for the recovery process come from the fibre itself and not from the applied stimulus. The stimulus merely acts as a trigger to release energy from the fibre.

In this period of relative refractoriness the spike height and the conduction velocity achieve complete recovery before the excitability does. Studies made with tetanising currents have shown that the refractory period of nerve is prolonged by re- peated stimuli and that both the oxygen consumption and the heat production fall, indicating an induced fatigue.

In work that has succeeded these fundamental observations of the pioneers, it has become clear that these periods of absolute and relative refractoriness have a basis in the ion transfers and resultant membrane polarisation levels following a propagated spike. As will become clearer in a subsequent chapter (Chapter 6), the inactivation of the sodium flux during the falling phase of the spike and the increased potassium influx to the neurone result in a level of depolarisation that cannot immediately generate another action potential.

The Supernormal Period. When the relatively refractory period gradually dies out the excitability of the nerve does not remain at the resting level but enters a period (lasting about 12 msec in A fibres) when it is more excitable, even by as much as 200 per cent above normal in excised nerves (7% *in vivo*), and can be readily induced to respond to a weaker stimulus than usual. The term 'supernormal' was applied to this phase by Adrian and Lucas, but it is probably more accurately regarded as a period of incomplete readjustment of the membrane potential after the conduction of an impulse. According to Gasser there is an increase in conduction velocity during this phase. Gasser has shown this period of heightened excitability to coincide with the negative after-potential. Both are increased in the presence of carbon dioxide.

The Subnormal Period. Graham, in 1935, was the first to demonstrate that following the phase of heightened excitability in nerve there is a subnormal period when the fibres are less readily excitable and the conduction velocity is impaired. In normal nerve, the time sequences of the excitability changes are found to resemble closely the duration of the different phases of the after-potentials (as can be seen in Fig. 16).

An interpretation of the excitability changes during sub-threshold stimulation of nerve is given in some detail in the discussion on electrotonic potentials in the section on stimulation of nerve by applied electric currents (see page 79).

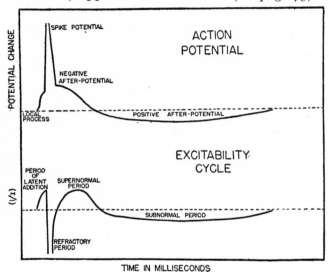

TIME IN MILLISECONDS

FIG. 16. THE ACTION POTENTIAL AND EXCITABILITY CYCLE OF A
TYPICAL SENSORY NEURONE

For diagrammatic purposes the duration of the first two phases of each
curve has been exaggerated.

(From Morgan (1943) *Physiological Psychology*, McGraw-Hill.)

The decrease in excitability during the subnormal period was at one time thought to have different characteristics from that of the relatively refractory period, since the spike is not reduced in size but the conduction velocity is slowed. Later work, however, suggests that these two periods are part of the same event, and that the subnormal period is a late continuation of the relatively refractory period which has been interrupted by the supernormal phase. The curve recorded is thus the algebraic sum of these events. This kind of depressed excitability is an impairment of the spike generating mechanism resulting from long-sustained depolarisation of the nerve membrane.

The excitability of nerve is very much influenced by repetition of the stimulus, a fact of some importance since this resembles the situation in the living animal more closely than does the isolated shock. Fatigue, even in a short and rapid

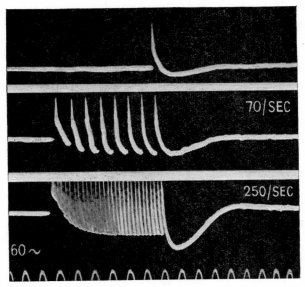

FIG. 17. INCREASE IN POSITIVE AFTER-POTENTIAL PRODUCED BY A SHORT TETANUS. A FIBRES OF THE PHRENIC NERVE (CAT)

The records start with the negative after-potential, for the spikes extend far beyond the tops of the records. The top record shows the result of a single shock; the centre record the result of a short tetanus at 70/sec, and the lowest record a tetanus of similar duration but 250/sec.

(From Gasser (1939) *J. Neurophysiol.*, **2**, 361.)

tetanus, quickly and greatly prolongs the refractory phase, and hence also delays recovery. Repeated stimuli to a nerve have the effect of shortening the negative and increasing the positive after-potentials. This can be seen quite clearly in Fig. 17, which shows the result in a cat's nerve of applying repeated stimuli for a short time; in this illustration the spike potentials extend far beyond the records and therefore the first event to be seen is the negative after-potential, decreasing in duration as the stimuli increase in frequency. The increased positive potential is very noticeable; with a longer tetanus this increased positivity may be succeeded by another long-lasting positive phase such as is illustrated in Fig. 18. Within limits, the size of the positive after-potential increases with the frequency and duration of the tetanus. During all this time, which may be as long as five minutes, the nerve is in a state of depressed excitability, a state which, as Gasser suggests, may be the basis for

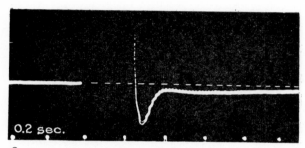

FIG. 18. AFTER-POTENTIALS IN THE PHRENIC NERVE OF THE CAT
AFTER A LONG TETANUS

The stimuli start at the break of the heavy line; the spikes go far beyond the record. The first visible tracing after the tetanus ends is the negative after-potential. This is followed by a large positive after-potential which, in its turn, is followed by a second positive deflection of long duration lasting beyond the limits of this record.

(From Gasser and Grundfest (1936) *Amer. J. Physiol.*, **117**, 113.)

some of the long-enduring changes in excitability found in the nervous system.

There is another relationship which emerges when one studies the excitability of different fibre types—the faster the conduction velocity the greater the excitability. In a mixed nerve trunk a stimulus may be graded in such a way that only the faster-conducting fibres respond. The resultant type of action potential will become clearer when the electrical response to a stimulus to a mixed nerve trunk has been studied (see Chapter 5).

Owing to the existence of a subnormal period it is possible to time stimuli to a nerve in such a way that they apparently inhibit nervous activity instead of exciting it. The first concept of this type of inhibition in peripheral nerve came from the experiments of Wedensky in 1884. He found that a muscle, moderately fatigued by stimulation through its motor nerve, reaches a stage when it fails to respond with more than a single initial contraction to stimulation impressed at a very high rate of repetition, although still responsive to slowly-repeated stimuli. The conditions for *Wedensky inhibition* in a nerve pathway in which there is a partial block of conduction at a synapse or neuro-muscular junction, are a series of stimuli so timed that each one after the first falls in the relatively refractory phase of its predecessor; the result is a series of subnormal impulses which are unable to pass the block. Such a block may be caused by drugs, pressure, cold or other agents (see page 59). The detailed work of Adrian and of Forbes has now clarified this subject. It is not a special type of fibre or a special type of impulse which produces this kind of inhibition rather than excitation, but solely the state of the fibre at the moment when it receives the stimulus.

A more complex type of inhibition is met with in the central nervous system, and this is described in Chapter 10.

BIBLIOGRAPHY

Adrian, E. D. (1913) Wedensky inhibition in relation to the 'all-or-none' principle in nerve. *J. Physiol. (Lond.)*, **46**, 384–412.

Adrian, E. D. (1920 and 1921) The recovery process in excitable tissues. *J. Physiol. (Lond.)*, **54**, 1–31 and **55**, 193–225.

Adrian, E. D. and Lucas, K. (1912) On the summation of propagated disturbances in nerve and muscle. *J. Physiol. (Lond.)*, **44**, 68–124.

Blair, H. A. (1939) Time constant of excitation and velocity in supernormal phase of nerve. *J. Neurophysiol.*, **2**, 249–255.

von Brücke, E. T., Early, M. and Forbes, A. (1941) Recovery of responsiveness in motor and sensory fibres during the relative refractory period. *J. Neurophysiol.*, **4**, 80–91.

Erlanger, J. and Gasser, H. S. (1937) *Electrical Signs of Nervous Activity*. University of Pennsylvania Press.

Forbes, A. (1934) 'A Mechanism of Reaction.' In *A Handbook of General Experimental Psychology*. Murchison. Clark University Press.

Gasser, H. S. (1936) Changes in nerve potentials produced by rapidly repeated stimuli and their relation to responsiveness of nerve to stimulation. *Amer. J. Physiol.*, **111**, 35–50.

Gasser, H. S. and Erlanger, J. (1925) Nature of conduction of impulse in relatively refractory period. *Amer. J. Physiol.*, **73**, 613–635.

Gasser, H. S. and Grundfest, H. (1936) Action and excitability in mammalian A fibres. *Amer. J. Physiol.*, **117**, 113–133.

Gotch, F. and Burch, C. J. (1899) The electrical response of nerve to two stimuli. *J. Physiol. (Lond.)*, **24**, 421–426.

Graham, H. T. (1936) The subnormal period of nerve response. *Amer. J. Physiol.*, **111**, 452–465.

Granit, R. and Phillips, C. G. (1956) Excitatory and inhibitory process acting upon individual Purkinje cells of the cerebellum in cats. *J. Physiol. (Lond.)*, **133**, 520–547.

Lucas, K. (1917) *The Conduction of the Nervous Impulse*. Longmans, London.

Rosenblueth, A., Alanis, J. and Mandoki, J. (1949) The functional refractory period of axons. *J. cell. comp. Physiol.*, **33**, 405–439.

Tasaki, I. (1949) The excitatory and recovery processes in the nerve fibre as modified by temperature changes. *Biochim. biophys. Acta, (Amst.)*, **3**, 498–509.

Tasaki, I. (1959) 'Conduction of the Nerve Impulse.' In *Handbook of Physiology—Neurophysiology*. Field, J., Magoun, H. W. and Hall, V. (Eds.). Vol. 1. American Physiological Society, Washington.

Wedensky, N. (1903) Die Erregung, Hemmung und Narkose. *Pflügers Arch. ges. Physiol.*, **100**, 1–144.

5

The Compound Action Potential of Nerve Trunks

IN a previous chapter we have seen the detailed potential changes accompanying a single nerve impulse in single fibres. In life, of course, these fibres run in tracts and form nerve trunks. Most of these nerve trunks are mixed, carrying fibres of more than one size and type which conduct impulses at various velocities. The action potential of such mixed nerves was studied in great detail by Erlanger and Gasser, and by Bishop and Heinbecker, who called it the compound action potential of nerve.

A single shock strong enough to stimulate all the fibres of a mixed nerve produces, at a distance from the site of stimulation, a train of electrical responses which at first glance seem to be of great complexity but which prove to have such constancy of character that their functions and relationships are now clearly understood.

On a descriptive level we may say that when there is an adequate length of nerve between the stimulating and recording electrodes there are three major complexes following a shock to a mixed nerve, *A*, *B* and *C*. The *A* complex which comes first and which is by far the largest consists of a large negative potential followed by a smaller one and then later by a still smaller one.

Erlanger and Gasser called these three components of the *A* complex by the Greek letters alpha, beta and gamma. Bishop, who was working with them at that time, rather irreverently calls this the neoclassical period, for the meaning of these elevations was at that time 'all Greek' to the group and, in fact, Gasser, years later, showed the gamma component to be an artefact. However, with this exception, these electrophysiologically defined elevations were shown by their discoverers to correlate extremely closely with fibre size as seen by the light microscope, and have therefore played a considerable part in neurophysiologists' understanding of the communication systems of the nervous system. They do not correlate with sensory modalities (such as touch, pain, heat and cold) as was originally hazarded as their function.

So much for the *A* complex. Following close on its heels comes the *B* complex, a single simpler elevation, followed in

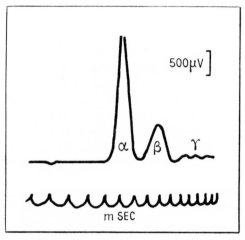

FIG. 19. THE *A* COMPLEX OF THE COMPOUND ACTION POTENTIAL OF A MIXED NERVE TRUNK RECORDED 13·1 CM FROM THE POINT OF STIMULATION

The full amplitude of the alpha elevation, which is the response of the largest fibres of the A group, is outside the limits of the record. The beta elevation is the response of the less rapidly conducting fibres of the A group. Peroneal nerve of bull-frog. Time line: 1,000/sec.

(After Erlanger and Gasser (1937) *Electrical Signs of Nervous Activity*. University of Pennsylvania Press.)

turn, after a comparatively long interval, by a small long-lasting *C* elevation which finally dies away. That is the end, the last response to the original single shock. Fig. 20 is a record taken at an amplification great enough to show the *B* and *C* elevations. These follow at a considerable time interval after the *A* complex which is consequently not shown here. In Fig. 21 the whole sequence of potentials in the compound action potential of nerve has been reconstructed to demonstrate the relative sizes and time relationships of the *A*, *B*, and *C* complexes.

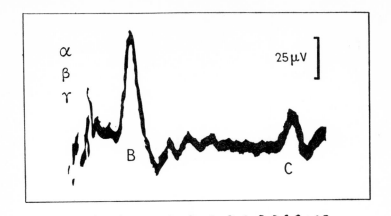

FIG. 20. THE *B* AND *C* ELEVATIONS OF THE COMPOUND ACTION
POTENTIAL OF A MIXED NERVE TRUNK

From the same nerve at the same conduction distance as in Fig. 19. The
A complex has preceded these elevations and is not shown here. Note the
great increase in amplification used in order to show these small elevations.
Time line: 60/sec.

(After Erlanger and Gasser (1937) *Electrical Signs of Nervous Activity.*
University of Pennsylvania Press.)

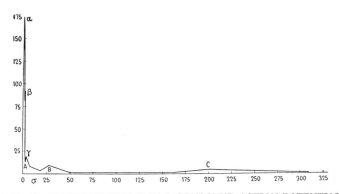

FIG. 21. RECONSTRUCTION OF A COMPOUND ACTION POTENTIAL

This demonstrates the relative sizes and time-relationships of the various
components. The *A* spike with its alpha and beta elevations is contributed
by the fibres of the A group, the *B* elevation by the slower-conducting
fibres of the B group, and the *C* elevation by the slowest of all the fibres.
Sciatic nerve of the bull-frog.

(From Erlanger and Gasser (1937) *Electrical Signs of Nervous Activity.*
University of Pennsylvania Press.)

45

Leaving the descriptive level of discussion, what do these elevations mean and what is responsible for their time relationships? Erlanger and Gasser demonstrated with great clarity that each of the several complexes is the response of a different type of fibre in the mixed nerve, the A fibres with the highest

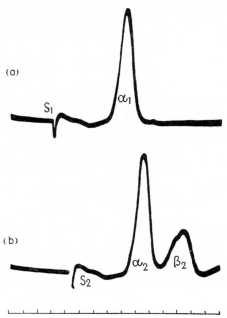

FIG. 22. COMPOUND ACTION POTENTIAL OF A NERVE TRUNK

Showing results from: (a) A stimulus strong enough to stimulate only the larger A fibres of low threshold. The upper curve shows the alpha elevation only. (b) A stronger stimulus evoking a response not only from these large fibres but from those of lesser diameter also. The lower curve shows the alpha elevation followed by beta elevation. Sciatic nerve of bull-frog. Time in msec.

(From Erlanger and Gasser (1937) *Electrical Signs of Nervous Activity.* University of Pennsylvania Press.)

conduction velocity being responsible for the alpha elevation, with a falling off through the whole range of conduction velocities to the slowest which produce their electrical response in the C elevation.

One of the critical proofs that these various elevations are the response of different fibre groups is given by the fact that a stimulus too weak to stimulate the smaller and less excitable fibres, for example the smaller A fibres responsible for the beta elevation, will evoke a response from the larger A fibres only, the resultant compound action potential showing an alpha elevation only. This point is illustrated in Fig. 22. It shows the

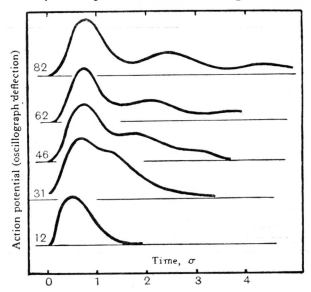

FIG. 23. COMPOUND ACTION POTENTIAL AFTER PROPAGATION
THROUGH VARYING DISTANCES

Cathode-ray oscillograph records, transferred to rectilinear co-ordinates, of the action current in a bull-frog's sciatic nerve, after propagation from the site of stimulation through the distances shown in mm on the left. At a distance 12 mm from the stimulus all are more or less together, but as the distance increases the small fibres of slower conduction rates respond later.

(From Erlanger and Gasser (1937) *Electrical Signs of Nervous Activity*. University of Pennsylvania Press.)

response of a nerve composed of A fibres of different conduction velocities to single shocks. In the upper curve the stimulus is too weak to evoke a response from any but the largest fibres of greatest excitability: it shows the alpha elevation only. In the lower curve the stimulus has been increased until less excitable fibres also respond and the beta elevation is evoked as well.

Hence the apparently complex compound action potential turns out to be the series responses of the fastest conducting and most excitable A fibres of large diameter (alpha elevation), followed by the slower conducting A fibres of lesser diameter (beta elevation), then by the smaller B fibres (*B* elevation) and finally by the very slowly conducting fine fibres of low excitability, the C fibres. All start out together at the point of stimulation but the impulses in each type of fibre become spatially

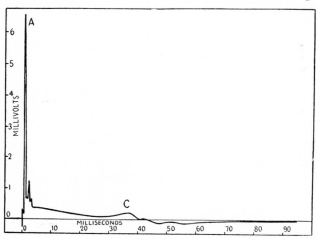

FIG. 24. SCHEMATIC REPRESENTATION OF THE COMPOUND ACTION
POTENTIAL OF THE SAPHENOUS NERVE OF THE CAT

The *A* complex contributed by the afferent fibres of the A type is seen in both amplitude and time relationship in the C elevation contributed by the slowly-conducted fibres of the C group.

(From Gasser (1938) *J. appl. Phys.*, **9**, 88.)

separated and reach a distant electrode in the order of their conduction velocities. The fastest one wins the race and the rest come tagging along behind. This race is illustrated in Fig. 23. At a point 12 mm from the start they are all neck-and-neck. At 31 mm the alpha components are pulling out ahead. At 82 mm they are far ahead.

In a mixed nerve then, if all the fibres are stimulated the shape of the compound action potential will be determined by the number of fibres of each type and conduction velocity present. The resultant whole is the aggregate of the parts. If the stimulus is not strong enough to excite all fibres the resultant compound action potential will have a different curve owing to

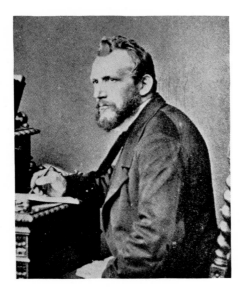

PLATE I

Emil Du Bois-Reymond (1818–1896)
who first demonstrated the action potential of nerve

'If I do not greatly deceive myself', he said, 'I have succeeded in realising in full actuality (albeit under a slightly different aspect) the hundred-years' dream of physicists and physiologists, to wit, the identity of the nervous principle with electricity.'

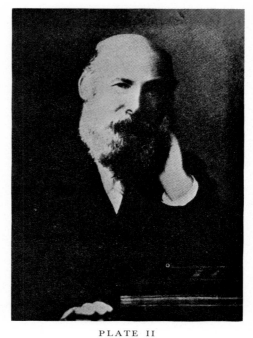

PLATE II

Julius Bernstein (1839–1917)

Formulator of the 'membrane theory' for nerve. (*Pflüger's Arch. ges. Physiol.*, (1902) **92,** 521) different levels of excitability of the various fibre types; A fibres having a lower threshold of response than B fibres; and B lower than C. As can be seen in Fig. 24, a mixed nerve having A and C fibres but no B fibres (such as the saphenous nerve of the cat) will give a compound action potential showing *A* and *C* elevations, but no *B* elevation. In this figure the very high *A* elevation was contributed by fibres whose conduction velocity was approximately 80 m/sec, and the low *C* elevation, occurring much later, by fibres with velocities of about 2 m/sec.

BIBLIOGRAPHY

Bishop, G. H. (1965) My life among the axons. *Ann. Rev. Physiol.*, **27,** 1–18.

Erlanger, J. (1927) The interpretation of the action potential in cutaneous and muscle nerves. *Amer. J. Physiol.*, **82,** 644–655.

Erlanger, J. and Gasser, H. S. (1937) *Electrical Signs of Nervous Activity*. University of Pennsylvania Press.

Gasser, H. S. (1928) The relation of the shape of the action potential of nerve to conduction velocity. *Amer. J. Physiol.*, **84,** 699–711.

Gasser, H. S. (1937) The control of excitation in the nervous system. *Harvey Lect.*, **32,** 169–193.

Gasser, H. S. (1935) Conduction in nerves and fibre types. *Res. Publ. Assoc. Res. nerv. ment. Dis.*, **15,** 35–39.

Gasser, H. S. (1950) Unmedullated fibres originating in dorsal root ganglia. *J. gen. Physiol.*, **33,** 651–690.

Gasser, H. S. (1958) Comparison of the structure, as revealed with the electron microscope, and the physiology of the unmedullated fibres in the skin nerves in the olfactory nerves. *Exp. Cell Res. Suppl.*, **5,** 3–17.

Gasser, H. S. and Erlanger, J. (1926) The role played by the sizes of the constituent fibres of a nerve trunk in determining the form of its action potential wave. *Amer. J. Physiol.*, **80,** 522–547.

Gasser, H. S. and Erlanger, J. (1929) The role of fibre size in the establishment of a nerve block by pressure or cocaine. *Amer. J. Physiol.*, **88,** 581–591.

Gasser, H. S. and Grundfest, H. (1939) Axon diameters in relation to spike dimensions and conduction velocity in mammalian fibres. *Amer. J. Physiol.*, **127,** 393–414.

Heinbecker, P., O'Leary, J. and Bishop, G. H. (1933) Nature and source of fibres contributing to the saphenous nerve of the cat. *Amer. J. Physiol.*, **104,** 23–35.

Hursh, J. B. (1939) Conduction velocity and diameter of nerve fibres. *Amer. J. Physiol.*, **127,** 131–139.

6

The Propagation of the Nerve Impulse

THE great communication systems of the body which enable it to react appropriately to both external and internal stimulation rely on the passage of impulses along nerves. The details of the mechanisms by which these messages are transmitted have been the subject of intense exploration ever since it was first recognised that the nerve impulse is identifiable with an electrical change. The unequivocal demonstration of the electrical potential of nerve by Du Bois-Reymond in the 1840s gave the death-blow to the vitalist's concept of 'animal spirits' as the activator of sensation and movement, and provided a restitution of Galvani's belief in animal electricity.

The travelling nerve impulse consists of a progression of ionic changes which derive the energy for their transmission from the metabolism of the nerve itself and not from the stimulus. There have been many hypotheses about this travelling wave of excitation, almost all of which derive from Bernstein's membrane theory, originally framed for the muscle fibre but subsequently applied to nerve. There can be no disagreement that this classical theory has made a useful working hypothesis even if the most recent work in this field is at variance with its acceptance without some modification and extension.

THE RESTING POTENTIAL

In 1902, Bernstein, following Ostwald's original concept, advanced the theory that the membrane of the inactive fibre is normally polarised, having positive ions on the outside and negative ions on the inside, and that the action potential is a self-propagating depolarisation of this membrane. This was based on his assumption that the membrane of the fibre is selectively permeable to potassium ions, and on the fact that a greater concentration (by about 20 : 1, or in some cases as much

as 65 : 1) is always present inside the resting uninjured fibre
than outside it.

If, without applying a stimulus, a suitable recording instrument is attached to two electrodes on the surface of a resting
nerve fibre, no current flows through the instrument. When,
however, the nerve is cut, the injured end becomes negative to
the rest of the fibre's surface and a current now flows in an
external circuit towards the cut end. This is exactly similar to
the currents of injury observed in muscle by the Italian scientist
Matteucci over a hundred years ago. In terms of the membrane
theory the explanation of this current of injury, or demarcation
current, is that the insulation between the inside of the nerve
and the outside environment has now been broken down and
potential difference at the membrane surface can no longer be
maintained. There is, as it were, a 'short-circuit' and current
flows in through the break in the membrane. The potential
difference of the demarcation potential of a neurone may be
as high as 50 mV, or even 90 mV depending on the type of
nerve.

This demarcation potential is detectable not only at the site
of the cut but also along the length of the nerve, decaying with increasing distance from the injury. This is illustrated in Fig. 25
which represents horizontally a nerve (N) injured at the point
h. At the point h the demarcation potential is at its maximum
and then falls away as shown by the curve; the lines of current
flow consistent with such a curve are shown below it.

To determine directly the resting potential of a single fibre
is technically difficult because of the size, but it was first done
in the giant nerve fibre of the squid, the largest known axon,
being about 500μ in diameter whereas the largest fibres in man
are not more than 10μ.

Hodgkin and Huxley inserted a microelectrode into the
axoplasm of one of these fibres so that its tip was opposite and
across the membrane from a second electrode on the outside of
the wall. A photograph of the electrode in place is reproduced
in Fig. 26. They found a potential difference in the resting
nerve of approximately 50 mV (inside the membrane being
negative to the outside) a value of the same order as that found
for the demarcation potential. Furthermore they were able to
demonstrate that this potential difference could be reduced to

zero by increasing the potassium ion concentration on the outside of the fibre by about 18 times the normal value. Very
similar techniques were also being used by Cole and Curtis at
this time with the same results.

Since this pioneer work on recording from within the axon,
microelectrode techniques have been developed for penetrating
and recording intracellular potentials from the cell bodies of

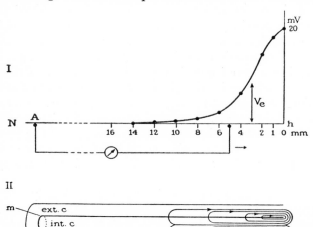

FIG. 25. DEMARCATION POTENTIAL OF A NERVE

A nerve, *N*, has been injured at the point *h*. The demarcation potential,
V_e, falls off with increasing distance from the injury. The lower diagram
represents the lines of current flow resulting from the break in the membrane
at the site of the injury. *m* represents the membrane; *int. c* the inside of the
nerve; *ext. c* the external medium.

(From Lorente de Nó (1947) *Harvey Lect.*, **42**, 43.)

neurones. This was first achieved in mammalian cell bodies of
the large motor neurones of the spinal cord which are only
some 70μ in diameter. In their earlier work, Eccles and his
colleagues used, as electrodes, glass capillaries filled with an
electrolyte and with a tip diameter of 0.5μ. Many types of even
finer electrodes have since been developed by many workers
throughout the world. In spinal motor neurones of the cat,
Eccles found the difference in potential across the membrane
to lie in a range of 60 to 80 μV. A similar order of transmembrane potential has been found for many cells (e.g. sympathetic

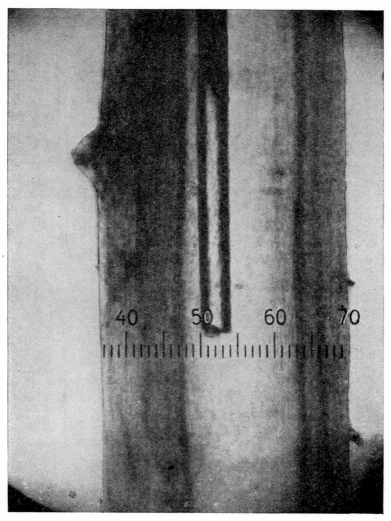

FIG. 26. PHOTOMICROGRAPH OF A RECORDING ELECTRODE INSIDE
A GIANT AXON OF A SQUID

This was used by Hodgkin and Huxley to measure the potential across the
nerve membrane. Each division of the scale equals 33 microns.
(From Hodgkin and Huxley (1945) *J. Physiol.* (*Lond.*), **104,** 176.)

ganglion cells, pyramidal cells in the cortex, and crustacean stretch receptor cells). There is evidence also that in a given neurone the membrane potential of the axon is the same as that of its parent cell.

The increase in external potassium and the depolarisation of the membrane do not, however, parallel each other exactly in time relations. Since potassium ions can, in fact, pass through the membrane, the fact that in resting nerve they have a higher concentration inside the membrane raises the basic question: what maintains the resting potential of the nerve fibre?

Bernstein held that the resting potential was maintained by the difference in concentration of potassium ions on either side of a membrane selectively impermeable to anions. According to such a hypothesis the membrane potential would be proportional to the logarithm of the ratio of the internal to the external concentration of potassium.* Although experimental data have been brought forward by several workers to support this relationship, it has been challenged by others. For example, Lorente de Nó's experiments on frog's nerve in potassium-free media in which he demonstrated that a nerve depolarised by lack of oxygen could be completely repolarised by restoring the oxygen supply, led him to the conclusion that the mechanism for creating and maintaining the resting potential (in contrast to the action potential) was oxidative metabolism. These conclusions have been challenged by some workers with the suggestion that some part of these effects may be due to characteristics of the connective tissue sheath of the nerve (epineurium).

An alternative hypothesis is that the resting potential is not due to the barrier of a semipermeable membrane between the oppositely charged ions but that it is an electrostatic potential: a double layer of oppositely charged ions held apart by the

---

* The Nernst equation is:

$$E = 0 \cdot 058 \log \frac{K_2}{K_1} \text{ V}$$

where E = potential difference,
    K_1 = potassium concentration inside the fibre,
    K_2 = potassium concentration of surrounding medium,
    $0 \cdot 058$ = the factor of proportionality at 18°C (frog).
Although many workers have evidence suggesting a linear relationship between E and $\log \frac{K_2}{K_1}$ the full calculated value for E has not been found experimentally for nerve membrane.

greater chemical affinity of the external medium for the positive ions, and the greater chemical affinity of the internal substance for the negative ions.

Other theories have been advanced to explain the resting membrane potential, one being that it is a phase-boundary potential across the lipoid membrane separating the aqueous axoplasm from the aqueous medium surrounding the nerve. This theory had its origins in the concept of Nernst.

However, the theory that has received the most general acceptance is that of Hodgkin and Huxley, for it meets the most criteria imposed by experimental observation. These workers have expressed this theory in the form of a mathematical model in which the distribution of membrane current along the axon is described by a partial differential equation and the non-linear current-voltage characteristics of the membrane by subsidiary differential equations.

THE ACTION POTENTIAL

According to the membrane theory, in the uninjured fibre when an impulse passes, the selective permeability of the membrane increases, producing a change in ionic flux; this results in a local inward flow of current from the outside of the nerve at the point of excitation (see Fig. 29). The outward flow of current in the surrounding extrapolar regions is what has been called 'catelectrotonus'. The current flows to the active point from an inactive part of the fibre to neutralise the charge, and this action in turn releases, at this new point, negative ions from inside the membrane to come out and repeat the process in the next portion of the fibre. The analogy to the travelling wave of electro-chemical activity in Lillie's model of an iron wire coated with oxide and immersed in nitric acid is famous. However, such a simple depolarisation as is suggested by this model would be inadequate to account for the observed data and this view is no longer tenable. The action spike is not merely a depolarisation of a previously-charged membrane. The mechanism of impulse propagation cannot be explained as a simple outflow of potassium ions although evidence for a leakage of potassium during activity has been found by Cowan in crustacean nerve during a tetanus, and confirmed by Keynes using radioactive potassium, and in mammalian nerve by Arnett and

Wilde, among others. The ion of importance in the action potential, in contrast to the resting potential, is the sodium ion (see page 57).

A theory based on simple depolarisation as the source of the action potential would necessarily limit the voltage of the action spike to that of the resting potential or rather less, since even

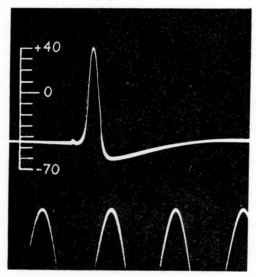

FIG. 27. ACTION POTENTIAL RECORDED BETWEEN INSIDE AND OUTSIDE OF AXON (SQUID NERVE)

The vertical scale indicates the potential of the internal electrode in mV, the sea water outside being taken as at zero potential. Time marker: 500 c/s.

(From Hodgkin and Huxley (1945) *J. Physiol. (Lond.),* **104,** 176.)

the depolarised membrane has some resistance. However, when Hodgkin and Huxley measured the action potential of squid nerve across the membrane of single fibres with a microelectrode inserted in the axoplasm they found it to be of higher voltage than the resting potential. Fig. 27 is a reproduction of Hodgkin and Huxley's record of an action potential recorded in this way. The resting potential in this case was minus 45 mV (inside negative to outside); at the passage of the impulse the action spike reached plus 40 mV, a total change of 85 mV (inside now positive to outside). A similar result was obtained by Cole and

Curtis; this is not peculiar to squid nerve, nor even to nerve, since muscle fibre has given the same result, and in recent years methods of penetrating nerve cell bodies have been developed that have confirmed this overshoot in mammalian neurones. In the original experiments the disparity between the voltage of the resting potential and of the action potential was thus found to be approximately 40 mV, an order of magnitude which was disturbing to the classical membrane theory of impulse propagation as it follows that the outside of the membrane must become negative to the inside at the moment of the action spike.

Various formulations have been advanced to account for this transitory reversal of potential. Höber drew attention to the possible role of organic anions, and an inductive element in the membrane reactance of squid nerve was suggested by Cole as a possible factor, but there is not yet evidence for this in vertebrate nerve. It seems well established that the difference in potassium ion concentration between the inside and the outside of the fibre, although an important factor, cannot be the sole explanation of the action potential. The clue is to be found in Hodgkin's work on the movement of sodium ions in squid nerve, for at the moment of excitation sodium enters the fibre through the membrane. Increasing the sodium concentration of the external medium increases the height of the action spike in squid axon, lowering the sodium reduces its height, and a sodium-free solution abolishes it altogether. The entry of sodium during activity has been confirmed in invertebrate nerve by Rothenburg and by Keynes, and in mammalian nerve by von Euler, all of whom used radioactive isotopes. Although sodium ions are apparently not essential for maintaining the resting potential, they are indispensable for maintaining the excitability of squid nerve.

Hodgkin's studies led to the formulation of a new hypothesis. Although the resting membrane is indeed, as Bernstein proposed, permeable to potassium yet almost impenetrable to sodium, it is postulated that this semipermeability reverses its preferential specificity during the rising phase of the action spike, allowing sodium to pass through more readily than either potassium or chloride. Thus, in an active nerve, when the external eddy currents flow into the fibre at the site of activity, sodium ions enter the membrane. A rapid movement of this kind would account for the reversal in potential. Hodgkin and Katz make the suggestion that the sodium may not cross the membrane in ionic form but that it may combine with a lipoid-soluble carrier made available by the depolarisation of the membrane; this proposal awaits proof but the experimental determination of the correlation between sodium concentration of the external medium and action potential in squid axon has given strong support to the main hypothesis which may be regarded as the most adequate of the many which have as yet been advanced to explain the action potential.

Movement of ions across a permeable membrane can occur freely by diffusion provided the electro-chemical gradient does not oppose it. However, in the recovery phase after the action potential the outward movement of sodium ions has to be forced against a gradient; this implies a pumping action, the energy for which would have to be derived from metabolic processes in the nerve. Though there is no direct proof of such a 'sodium pump', the hypothesis covers most of the experimental findings.

The theory of electrical transmission of the nerve impulse is now generally accepted, the work from the Cambridge laboratory having done most to consolidate its standing. In its simplest form the theory states that transmission is effected by the excitatory action on adjacent inactive portions of the nerve by local circuits set up at the passage of an impulse by movement of ions across the membrane.

Evidence that eddy currents drawn to an active region of nerve fibre are able to increase the excitability of neighbouring parts was contributed in 1937 by Hodgkin, who studied, in the myelinated nerve of frog, the behaviour of the travelling nerve impulse on meeting a block. It is well known that the impulse can be blocked by many agents, such as drugs, cold, pressure, and by the depolarising action of an impressed electric current. When a cold or pressure block is made which extinguishes the propagated impulse, a potential change can be detected in the nerve beyond the area of the block; this potential change, called by Hodgkin the extrinsic potential, to distinguish it from the propagated action potential which initiated it, has been shown by him to have all the properties of a simple electrotonic potential such as is known to be set up in nerve when stimulated by electric currents (see page 79). Both the extrinsic potential and the electrotonic potential decay exponentially in time and in space. In other words, there is an outward flow of current, a catelectrotonus, which decreases the threshold of the fibre beyond the block that stopped the impulse. The presence of this catelectrotonic effect explains the observation made by Blair and Erlanger that, within time relations imposed by the conduction velocity of nerve, a subthreshold stimulus impressed beyond a block can sum with the eddy currents of a blocked impulse to evoke a response. It also explains the observation

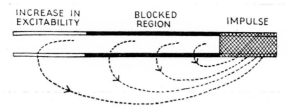

FIG. 28. SCHEMATIC DIAGRAM OF THE SPREAD OF THE EDDY
CURRENTS FROM AN IMPULSE THROUGH A BLOCKED REGION OF
NERVE

Transmission of the nerve impulse stops at the blocked region which cannot supply the energy for an action potential, but the local flow of the eddy current extends beyond the block by physical spread and increases the excitability of the region beyond the block. The impulse is travelling from right to left.

(From Hodgkin (1937) *J. Physiol. (Lond.)*, **90**, 183.)

that, if the blocked region be sufficiently small, the propagated impulse can jump the gap. Similarly, an action potential can be carried across a gap by a bridge made of any conducting material, such as, for example, a salt bridge. A schematic representation, taken from Hodgkin, of the passage of eddy currents through a blocked region of nerve is shown in Fig. 28.

Data of this kind support the electrical theory which is in essence a modification of the original core-conduction theory advanced by Hermann in 1879 (see Plate III, facing page 82). This pictured the nerve as a cylindrical tube consisting of an inner conducting core (the axoplasm) separated from an outer longitudinal conductor (the interstitial fluid and tissues) by a membrane having high resistance and some capacitance. When an impulse passes there will be a current flowing in one direction inside the fibre and in the other direction outside the fibre, and these eddy currents will act as an electrical stimulus on neighbouring stretches of inactive nerve.

Thus, as shown in the schematic drawing in the lower half of Fig. 29, there is, at the (shaded) active region, an inward flow or 'sink' of current (an electrotonus) which decreases the membrane potential, making it more permeable to sodium ions and internally electropositive, whereas the (unshaded) as yet

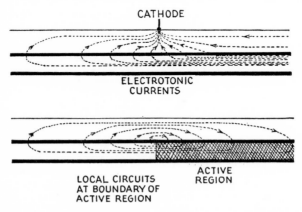

FIG. 29. SCHEMATIC DIAGRAM OF THE CURRENT FLOW RESPONSIBLE FOR ELECTROTONIC CURRENTS AND FOR THE NERVE IMPULSE

Above: On cathodal stimulation of a nerve. *Below:* Local circuits of a travelling nerve impulse.

(From Hodgkin (1937) *J. Physiol. (Lond.)*, **90**, 183.)

inactive part of the fibre is still permeable and electronegative. The current streams through the surrounding tissue into this sink from neighbouring inactive areas of the nerve which thus form 'sources'. The current coming out at these sources (catelectrotonus) acts as an electrical stimulus there, discharges the membrane and sets up a new locus of excitation. Schematic representations of these currents are shown in Fig. 29, which depicts the local circuits resulting from cathodal stimulation (above) and from local currents (below).

These ionic shifts are very transient (as transient as the nerve impulse itself) for immediately the impulse has passed by, the membrane resumes its previous permeability characteristics, potassium ions rush out of the fibre to restore the transmembrane balance and prepare the fibre for the passage of another impulse.

Added evidence for the importance to the action potential of potassium ions being concentrated at such a high ratio inside the fibre, has been supplied by the ingenious method developed by Baker and Shaw for extruding the axoplasm from squid giant axons and replacing it by known salts. Replacement by almost any salt of potassium was found to restore the action potential

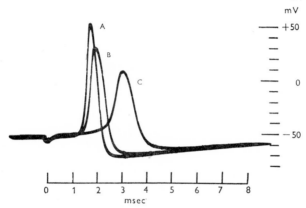

FIG. 30. EFFECT ON ACTION POTENTIAL OF REPLACING INTERNAL
POTASSIUM WITH SODIUM IONS

A, isotonic potassium sulphate; *B*, ¼K replaced by Na; *C*, ½K replaced
by Na.

(From Baker, Hodgkin and Shaw (1961) *Nature*, **190**, 885.)

of the fibre, the nature of the anion being apparently unimportant. The essential requirement is the establishment of a potassium ion gradient.

If the axoplasm is replaced by a mixture of potassium and sodium salts the action potential decreases in size with increasing proportions of sodium ions (as illustrated in Fig. 30) until total replacement of potassium by sodium abolishes the action potential entirely.

The discussion so far has described propagation of the nerve impulse in unmyelinated nerve, but in mammals the majority of fibres are myelinated (see page 3). In these nerves the local circuits flow from each Ranvier node to the next, for the intermediate sections, being covered by lipid material, have a very high impedance. The action currents developed at the exposed membrane of each node act as stimulating currents to the next node along the length of the fibre, the internodes acting as passive core conductors. Because in these nerves the impulse has to leap from node to node, this form of conduction has been named 'saltatory transmission'. Detailed studies of its characteristics will be found in the writing of Huxley and Stämpfli and of Tasaki.

If this cable-like structure is assumed for nerve, four electrical constants will be factors contributing to the behaviour of the fibre: the respective resistances of the axoplasm, the membrane and the external fluid, and the capacitance of the membrane.

It follows that if there is indeed a current flowing outside the fibre an increase of external resistance should slow the velocity of transmission. That this effect does take place has been demonstrated by Hodgkin. Single fibres of crab nerve conduct 14–40 per cent faster in seawater than in oil. Squid axons show an even greater difference; their conduction rate is 80–140 per cent faster in seawater than in either air or oil.

One of the observed effects in nerve which brings support to the theory of propagation by eddy currents is that an impulse travelling in one fibre can modify the excitability of adjacent fibres. Such an influence of activity in one fibre on its inactive neighbours was strongly suggested by the work of Adrian on injury discharges in mammalian fibres, and that of Hoagland on the synchronisation of impulses in the lateral line nerves of fish. This has since been demonstrated in crab nerve, in squid and in toad by many workers, among whom are Jasper and Monnier, Katz and Schmitt, Arvanitaki, and Tasaki. The technique used by Jasper and Monnier was to juxtapose two groups of unmyelinated fibres for a distance of about 1 cm and then apply a chemical stimulus to one group only. In those cases where the adjacent resting nerve was on the verge of spontaneous rhythmic discharge (that is, when it was highly excitable), transmission took place at the site of contact after a long delay (about 20 msec).

Katz and Schmitt took this work further by using single fibres, again from unmyelinated crab nerve. They found mutual interaction between two adjacent fibres which was both qualitatively and quantitatively in keeping with the hypothesis of eddy currents flowing outside the active fibre and penetrating the resting fibre. Figure 31 shows schematically the local circuits and demonstrates that whereas at the site of the action potential in the active fibre there is a sink of current flanked by two sources (such as is studied in detail in Chapter 7), in the receiving fibre there is a source flanked by two sinks. The effect of this is at first to lower the excitability of the receiving fibre,

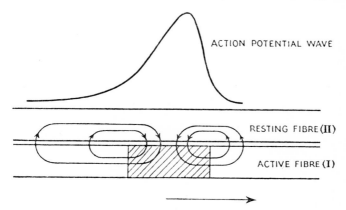

FIG. 31. PENETRATION OF A RESTING FIBRE (II) BY AN ACTION CURRENT IN THE ACTIVE FIBRE (I)

Spatial distribution of voltage is shown in the upper part of the figure. (From Katz and Schmitt (1939–1940) *J. Physiol. (Lond.)*, **97**, 471.)

then raise it and then lower it again. This sequence of excitability changes, as determined experimentally, is shown in Fig. 32. In every case these effects are subliminal, that is, they are below the threshold to initiate an impulse in the second fibre, but of course they have an important facilitating effect on any other activity in the fibre. It has been calculated that less than one-third of the external current of the active fibre actually penetrates the receiving fibre owing to the impedance of the membranes, interstitial fluid and possible connective tissue between them.

Arvanitaki, however, using squid nerve was able to produce a propagated impulse in the receiving fibre in an experimental setting in which she made an artificial synapse between the two fibres. This she called an 'ephapse'. The response in the receiving fibre was sufficient to initiate an impulse only when it had been sensitised by decalcification (by citrate).

As long ago as 1859, Pflüger observed that the excitability of nerves can be increased at the cathode during the passage of a constant current. Rosenblueth has used this method to heighten the excitability of myelinated fibres in cat's nerve,

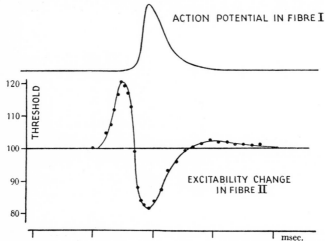

FIG. 32. EXCITABILITY CHANGES IN A RESTING FIBRE CAUSED BY THE PASSAGE OF AN ACTION POTENTIAL IN AN ADJACENT FIBRE

The time course is shown in the upper part of the figure. The threshold in the resting fibre is at first raised, then lowered, and then again raised.
(From Katz and Schmitt (1939–1940) *J. Physiol. (Lond.)*, **97**, 471.)

and in this way has been able to stimulate resting fibres by the passage of nerve impulses in adjacent active ones.

These data, obtained from isolated nerve in artificial settings, make it seem unlikely that action potentials in the nervous system actually initiate propagated impulses in neighbouring fibres, but it is strong evidence that they may facilitate them. The role of this mechanism as a synchronising agent in rhythmic nervous activity is discussed in a later section.

The theory just described for electrical propagation of the nerve impulse, although it includes several as yet unproven assumptions, receives more general acceptance than its major rival of a few years ago. This laid emphasis on chemical reactions involving acetylcholine. It owed its development mainly to

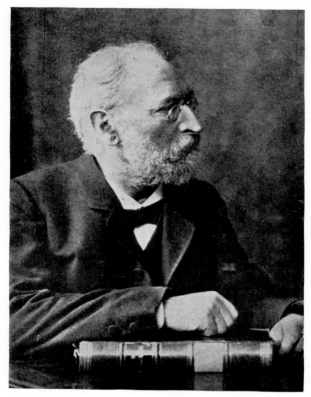

PLATE III

Ludimar Hermann (1838–1914)
The first to define with clarity the demarcation potential of nerve.

Below is a schema suggested by him for the nerve impulse. It is interesting
to compare this with Fig. 29.

(Photograph reproduced by courtesy of Professor H. Lullies of Kiel)

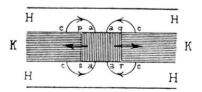

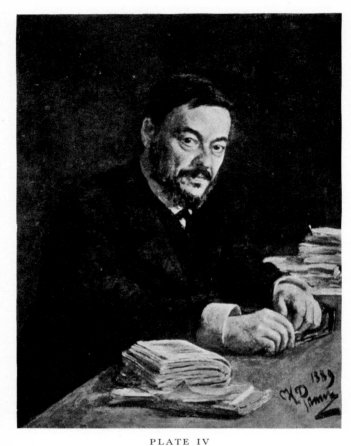

PLATE IV

Ivan Michailovich Sechenov (1829–1905)

First of the great Russian physiologists and a pioneer in studies of the electrical activity of the spinal cord and medulla.

(*From the portrait by Repin in the Tretyakov Gallery, Moscow*) the work of Nachmansohn who postulated that flow of current in local circuits is the agent for transmission of the impulse along the fibre, but that depolarisation is dependent for its development on the chemical mediation of acetylcholine. According to this hypothesis the depolarisation accompanying the passage of the impulse results from a fall in membrane resistance following an increase in permeability caused by the sudden appearance of acetylcholine released by the flow of current out of the inactive region. Repolarisation would depend on the very rapid destruction of acetylcholine by the enzyme cholinesterase, which is present in the membrane. Nachmansohn considers that these chemical changes can take place with a rapidity adequate for the time characteristics of the action potential, though this has been challenged.

Supporting evidence for the second part of this theory (restoration of polarisation by inactivation of acetylcholine) is the high concentration of cholinesterase found in nervous tissue; the relative specificity of cholinesterase in hydrolysing acetylcholine; the localisation of this enzyme exclusively to the surface of the nerve fibre (at least in squid nerve); and the fact that the action potential is abolished if the cholinesterase is inhibited (for example, by a strong concentration of eserine). The role of acetylcholine is inferred from the distribution and properties of the enzyme.

On the other hand, opponents of a universal theory for chemical transmission mediated by acetylcholine emphasise that the amounts of this substance synthesised by sensory nerves as, for example, the optic nerves or the dorsal spinal roots or by postganglionic fibres of sympathetic nerves, are too small to be allotted so important a role.

All theories, however, recognise the occurrence of a drop in resistance across the membrane as a crucial event in the passage of the impulse. This was first demonstrated by Cole and Curtis in the giant axon of the squid, where they found a transient fall in membrane resistance from $1,000 \ \Omega/cm^2$ of membrane area to 25 during the passage of the impulse. The resistance of the membrane may be regarded as an index of the ion permeability of the membrane.

In the motor neurone of the mammalian spinal cord Eccles found a membrane resistance in the order of $400 \ \Omega/cm^2$. Cole

6—(B.B.23)

and Curtis found a capacitance value of about $1\mu\mathrm{F}/\mathrm{cm}^2$ for the membrane of squid nerve, a value of the same order as that found for many other biological membranes. A somewhat higher figure for the capacitance of mammalian motor neurones is suggested by the work of Eccles and his group. Unlike the resistance, the capacitance of the nerve membrane scarcely changes during the passage of an impulse.

Opposing theories of transmission of the nerve impulse once formed one of the outstanding controversies in nerve physiology, a neurohumoral school and an electrical school each having its adherents. In fact, so general was the controversy at one time that it was often irreverently referred to as the 'battle between the soup and the sparks'. But, as will be seen from the account above, there is now a common meeting ground in the general acceptance of propagation by local currents, the issue that is still controversial being whether or not acetylcholine plays a role in the process.

BIBLIOGRAPHY

Arvanitaki, A. (1942) Effects evoked in an axon by the activity of a contiguous one. *J. Neurophysiol.*, **5**, 89–108.

Baker, P. F., Hodgkin, A. L. and Shaw, T. I. (1962) Replacement of the protoplasm of a giant nerve fibre with artificial solutions. *J. Physiol. (Lond.)*, **164**, 330–354.

Baker, P. F. (1965) Phosphorus metabolism of intact crab nerve and its relation to the active transport of ions. *J. Physiol. (Lond.)*, **180**, 383–423.

Bernstein, J. (1912) *Elektrobiologie*. Vieweg, Brunswick.

Bishop, G. H. (1956) Natural history of the nerve impulse. *Physiol. Rev.*, **36**, 376–399.

Caldwell, P. C. and Keynes, R. D. (1960) The permeability of the squid giant axon to radioactive potassium and chloride ions. *J. Physiol. (Lond.)*, **154**, 177–189.

Cole, K. S. and Baker, R. F. (1941) Longitudinal impedance of the squid giant axon. *J. gen. Physiol.*, **24**, 771–788.

Cole, K. S. and Curtis, H. J. (1939) Electric impedance of the squid giant axon during activity. *J. gen. Physiol.*, **22**, 649–670.

Davson, H. and Danielli, J. F. (1943) *Permeability of Natural Membranes*. Cambridge University Press, London.

Du Bois-Reymond, R. *Untersuchungen über Thierische Electricität*. Vol. 1, 1848; Vol. 2, 1849. Reimer, Berlin.

Eccles, J. C. (1957) *The Physiology of Nerve Cells.* Johns Hopkins Press, Baltimore.

Eyzaguirre, C. and Kuffler, S. W. (1955) Further study of soma, dendrites and axon excitation in single neurones. *J. gen. Physiol.*, **39**, 121–153.

Frankenheuser, B. (1960) Quantitative description of sodium currents in myelinated nerve fibres of *Xenopus laevis*. *J. Physiol. (Lond.)*, **151**, 491–501.

Hebb, C. O. (1954) Acetylcholine metabolism of nervous tissue. *Pharmacol. Rev.*, **6**, 39–43.

Hermann, L. (1899) Zur Theorie der Erregungsleitung und der electrischen Erregung. *Pflügers Arch. ges. Physiol.*, **75**, 574–590.

Hess, A. and Young, J. Z. (1949) Correlation of internodal length and fibre diameter in the central nervous system. *Nature*, **164**, 490–491.

Hodgkin, A. L. (1937) Evidence for electrical transmission in nerve. *J. Physiol. (Lond.)*, **90**, 183–232.

Hodgkin, A. L. (1939) The relation between conduction velocity and the electrical resistance outside a nerve fibre. *J. Physiol. (Lond.)*, **94**, 560–570.

Hodgkin, A. L. (1947) The membrane resistance of a non-medullated nerve fibre. *J. Physiol. (Lond.)*, **106**, 305–318.

Hodgkin, A. L. (1947) The effect of potassium on the surface membrane of an isolated axon. *J. Physiol. (Lond.)*, **106**, 319–340.

Hodgkin, A. L. (1951) The ionic basis of electrical activity in nerve and muscle. *Biol. Rev.*, **26**, 339–401.

Hodgkin, A. L. (1958) Ionic movements and electrical activity in giant nerve fibres. *Proc. roy. Soc. B.*, **148**, 1–37.

Hodgkin, A. L. (1964) *The Conduction of the Nervous Impulse.* C. C. Thomas, Springfield.

Hodgkin, A. L. and Huxley, A. F. (1945) Resting and action potentials in single nerve fibres. *J. Physiol. (Lond.)*, **104**, 176–195.

Hodgkin, A. L. and Huxley, A. F. (1947) Potassium leakage from an active nerve fibre. *J. Physiol. (Lond.)*, **106**, 341–366.

Hodgkin, A. L. and Huxley, A. F. (1952) A quantitative description of membrane current and its application to conduction and excitation in nerve. *J. Physiol. (Lond.)*, **117**, 500–544.

Hodgkin, A. L. and Katz, B. (1949) The effect of sodium ions on the electrical activity of the giant axon of the squid. *J. Physiol. (Lond.)*, **108**, 37–77.

Hodgkin, A. L. and Keynes, R. D. (1955) Active transport of cations in giant axons from Sepia and Loligo. *J. Physiol. (Lond.)*, **128**, 28–60.

Hodgkin, A. L. and Keynes, R. D. (1956) Experiments on the injection of substances into squid giant axons by means of a microsyringe. *J. Physiol. (Lond.)*, **131**, 592–616.

Huxley, A. F. (1959) Ion movements during nerve activity. *Ann. N.Y. Acad. Sci.*, **81**, 221–246.

Huxley, A. F. and Stämpfli, R. (1949) Evidence for saltatory conduction in peripheral myelinated nerve fibres. *J. Physiol. (Lond.)*, **108**, 315–339.

Jasper, H. H. and Monnier, A. M. (1938) Transmission of excitation between excised non-myelinated nerves. An artificial synapse. *J. cell. comp. Physiol.*, **11**, 259–277.

Katz, B. and Schmitt, O. H. (1940) Excitability changes in a nerve fibre during the passage of an impulse in an adjacent fibre. *J. Physiol. (Lond.)*, **97**, 471–488.

Keynes, R. D. (1951) The ionic movements during nervous activity. *J. Physiol. (Lond.)*, **114**, 119–150.

Lorente de Nó, R. (1947) *A study of nerve physiology.* Monographs 131 and 132, Rockefeller Institute, New York.

Lorente de Nó, R. and Honrubia, V. (1965) Theory of the flow of action currents in isolated myelinated nerve fibres. *Proc. nat. Acad. Sci. (Wash.)*, **53**, 757–764, 938–945, 1384–1391; **54**, 82–89, 388–396, 770–777, 1061–1069, 1303–1310.

Nachmansohn, D. (1953–4) Metabolism and function of the nerve cell. *Harvey Lect.*, **49**, 57–99.

Pflüger, E. (1859) *Physiologie des Electrotonus.* Hirschwald, Berlin.

Rashbass, C. and Rushton, W. A. H. (1949) The relation of structure to the spread of excitation in the frog's sciatic trunk. *J. Physiol. (Lond.)*, **110**, 110–135.

Robertson, J. D. (1960) The molecular structure and contact relationships of cell membranes. *Progr. Biophys.*, **10**, 343–418.

Rushton, W. A. H. (1927) Effect upon the threshold for nervous excitation of the length of nerve exposed and the angle between current and nerve. *J. Physiol. (Lond.)*, **63**, 357–377.

Stämpfli, R. (1954) Saltatory conduction in nerve. *Physiol. Rev.*, **34**, 101–112.

Tasaki, I. (1953) *Nervous Transmission.* C. C. Thomas, Springfield.

Tasaki, I. (1959) 'Conduction of the Nerve Impulse.' In *Handbook of Physiology—Neurophysiology.* Vol. I. Field, J., Magoun, H. W. and Hall, V. (Eds.). American Physiological Society, Washington.

Tasaki, I., Singer, I. and Watanabe, A. (1965) Excitation of internally perfused squid giant axons in sodium-free media. *Proc. nat. Acad. Sci. (Wash.)*, **54**, 763–769.

7

The Electrical Field Around the Action Potential in a Conducting Medium

Iᴛ is essential for the physiologist when studying the electrical properties of nerve *in situ* to be able to distinguish the true electrical signs of active nerve from polarity changes imposed by the position and orientation of his recording electrodes. A nerve in its natural milieu lies embedded in tissue which is itself an electrolytic conductor, and therefore the shape of the action potential as recorded from the nerve in the body differs in many important respects from that of the artificial laboratory preparation in which the nerve is usually suspended on electrodes in air or in oil. The effect of a conducting medium on the record obtained has been most clearly set out by Bishop and O'Leary, and by Lorente de Nó. The most outstanding difference between the action potential recorded from the nerve in its natural environment as opposed to the laboratory specimen in its moist chamber is that the common form is triphasic rather than monophasic. In Fig. 33 an action potential in a non-conducting medium is illustrated for comparison with a similar recording from an isolated nerve in a conducting medium (cf. Fig. 9).

In an electrolytic conductor it is by the migration of ions that the current flows (anions to anode, cations to cathode) in contrast to a metallic conductor in which it is the movement of the electrons themselves that constitutes the current flow. As we have seen in Chapter 6 there is, as the impulse travels along the fibre, a flow of current into the nerve at the point of excitation, or in other words, a 'sink' of current or cathode. Cations are attracted to it, and at the moment of breakdown of membrane permeability sodium enters the nerve. At the same time there is an outward flow of current through the inactive but electrolytically conducting tissue on all sides of this active point, causing it to be, in terms of its environment, flanked by

69

'sources' of current to which anions are drawn. A schematic sketch of the potential changes due to the passage of a single impulse in a nerve in a conducting medium is shown in Fig. 34,

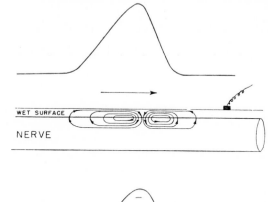

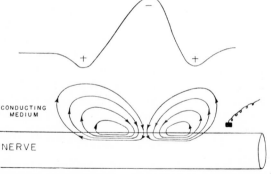

FIG. 33. COMPARISON BETWEEN ACTION POTENTIALS RECORDED IN
A NON-CONDUCTING MEDIUM (ABOVE) AND IN A VOLUME
CONDUCTOR (BELOW)

The nerve impulse is depicted as travelling towards an exploring electrode
on the wet surface of the nerve, the dimensions of which have been grossly
exaggerated for the purposes of demonstration.
The outlines of the monophasic (above) and triphasic action potentials
(below) are indicative of the changes in potential *in time* as recorded by
the electrode as the impulse approaches, arrives and departs.

in which certain dimensions have been grossly exaggerated for
diagrammatic purposes. When the nerve is at rest there is no
potential difference between the two electrodes. As can be seen
in section A of this diagram, the exploring electrode (the second
electrode being at a remote point in the conducting medium)

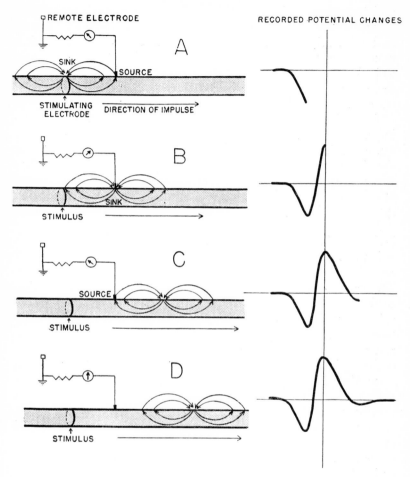

FIG. 34. SCHEMATIC DIAGRAM OF THE PASSAGE OF AN IMPULSE
ALONG A NERVE IN A CONDUCTOR MEDIUM

The exploring electrode is on the surface of the nerve, the second on
inactive tissue having the properties of an electrolytic conductor. The
resultant excursions of the recording instrument are shown on the right.

is, at the moment of stimulation to the nerve, over a source which attracts anions. The exploring electrode is, therefore, at this moment less negative than when the nerve was at rest and relatively positive to the far distant electrode, and thus causes a downward deflection in the recording instrument* such as is sketched to the right of the diagram. The direction of this deflection indicates the direction of change of potential difference, i.e. relative and not absolute polarity.

In section B the situation a moment later is shown when the impulse has travelled along the nerve and is now immediately underneath the exploring electrode. This electrode is now over the sink of the current, which is flowing in at this point so that this region is now negative to neighbouring areas of the nerve and to the tissue in which it is embedded. The recording system at this instant therefore registers an upward deflection.

In section C the impulse has passed along and the electrode is once again over a source, the sink into which the current flows being at a distant point along the fibre, leaving that part of the nerve under the electrode relatively positive to its environment. The record consequently shows a second downward deflection as the recording needle descends from the crest of the negative spike. Finally, in section D the impulse has passed by, the electrode is over resting nerve, and the recorded excursion has returned to the baseline. The relative duration and amplitude of the various components of the triphasic wave shown in section D of Fig. 34 will vary with the position of the recording electrode: the nearer it is to the stimulus the shorter the first positive phase.

It is interesting to compare the shape of the action potential of a nerve recorded thus in a conducting medium with the more common recording made from a nerve suspended in air or in oil, examples of which have been seen in Figs 10 and 11. The positive fields preceding and following the negative action spike are almost absent in a non-conducting medium. In a conducting medium the physical properties are of a field such as surrounds any electrical source in a similar medium. The distribution of the potential fields around a simple dipole are well known. Fig. 35 illustrates, in two dimensions only, a typical field around a source and sink of current such as is

* See footnote on p. 14.

found for any simple generator of electricity. The current flow (according to the traditional concept) is from the positive pole to the negative, and at right angles to the current flow are the contours of equal voltage. These are shown in this diagram as lines, but are, in a three-dimensional medium, surfaces of equipotential.

The schema in Fig. 36 made by Lorente de Nó for the field of the nerve action potential is the composite field of a pair of dipoles oriented longitudinally and in opposition, so that

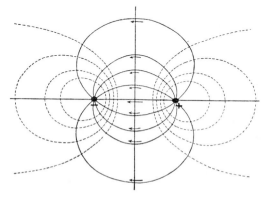

FIG. 35. DIAGRAM OF THE POTENTIAL FIELD AND CURRENT FLOW
ABOUT A DIPOLE IN A CONDUCTING MEDIUM
Isopotential contours are shown in broken lines, current flow in solid lines.
(From Lloyd (1955) *Howell's Textbook of Physiology.* Saunders.)

polarity is reversed at the site of action. His experimentally-determined fields for the action potential of bullfrog sciatic nerve gave just this distribution of voltage. In Fig. 36 is repre-sented the field he determined for the situation similar to that depicted in our Fig. 34 at the moment of time (*P*) as marked by the vertical line in each of the four curves at the bottom of this illustration. His technique was to lay a length of nerve on a piece of blotting paper soaked in Ringer solution (see sketch of lay-out at upper right of Fig. 36). The stimulated end of the nerve lay in a bath of mineral oil in a block of insulating material (see upper left of Fig. 36). The fields around the nerve were charted by locating with a finely-pointed exploring elec-trode the lines of equal potential. In a volume conductor the fields are, of course, three dimensional and the depicted lines should be thought of as surfaces. In Lorente de Nó's diagram,

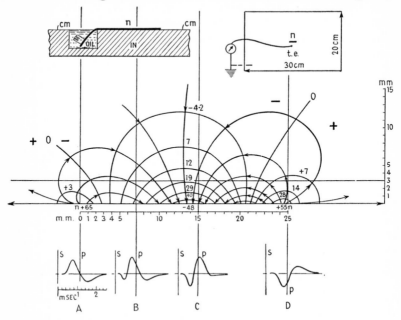

FIG. 36. THE FIELD OF CURRENT AROUND A NERVE IMPULSE

This field diagram was plotted at the moment in time marked by the line *p* in each of the curves from hundreds of positions of the recording electrode (see text). *S* represents the instant of stimulation in each case. In these two oppositely-oriented dipoles the two zero potential lines are marked *O* and are the curves without arrow-heads. All points lying between these zero lines are negative (i.e. sinks), those outside are positive (sources). *Upper left:* Nerve being stimulated in a bath of mineral oil, with the axon protruding out into a piece of blotting paper soaked in Ringer solution. *Upper right:* Plan of the blotting paper showing the nerve (*n*) lying in the centre, the exploring electrode (*t.e.*), and the remote electrode near the edge of the blotting paper.

(Redrawn from Lorente de Nó (1947) *A Study of Nerve Physiology*. Rockefeller Institute.)

reproduced here, only one-half of the field in a two-dimensional plane is shown.

The data from which he plotted these fields were obtained from hundreds of positions of the exploring electrode: four examples of these are given at the bottom of the figure. All four of these action potential curves, *A*, *B*, *C*, and *D*, were recorded from electrodes at a distance 3 mm from the nerve (see scale at the right of the diagram). The nerve is represented by the baseline. Curve *A* is the data obtained with a recording electrode opposite the point where the nerve entered the conducting medium. At the instant *P* the voltage is approximately zero in the curve *A*. In the diagram this is near to the zero potential line on the left and the line 3 mm from the nerve. In curve *B*, taken with a recording electrode 7 mm along the nerve, the recorded potential can be seen to be negative at the instant *P* and would fall in the field at approximately —9 (arbitrary units) and again 3 mm from the nerve. In curve *C*, when the electrode was 15 mm along the nerve, the experimentally found potential was strongly negative and is plotted in the field as —19. In curve *D* the electrode was on the end of the nerve and gave a positive potential plotted in the diagram as approximately + 7. Each of these points just referred to is plotted at the intersection of the straight line drawn 3 mm from the nerve and the projections of the straight line *P* in each of the four action potential curves, *A*, *B*, *C*, and *D*.

The rest of the field was plotted from other positions of the exploring electrode, both nearer and farther from the nerve than the set of data detailed here. The final map shows a sink of current flanked by two sources; the action potential shows a negative phase flanked by two positive ones.

The shape of a recorded action potential of a nerve in a conducting medium is determined by the position and orientation of the recording electrodes. At the same moment in time, the action potential recorded at different points along the nerve has a different shape. This is illustrated more fully in Figs 37 and 38, which reproduce Lorente de Nó's data. Figure 37 shows the recorded action potential from the following positions of the electrode: *A*, at the point where the nerve enters the conducting field; *B*, 7 mm along the nerve; *C*, 15 mm; and *D*, 26 mm along the nerve and at its end. Increasing the distance between the stimulating electrodes and the recording electrode has a marked effect on the shape of the curve obtained. Position *A*, being at the edge of the conducting medium, does not record the approach of the travelling impulse, only its occurrence and departure. Position *B* records some of its approach; position *C* more. Position *D* being at the end of the nerve cannot receive current flow from a section ahead of it and therefore records no second positive swing. Neither *A* nor *D* can be regarded as situations having parallels in the living animal.

Figure 38, in contrast, demonstrates the influence on the recorded wave-form of increasing the distance between the recording electrode and the surface of the nerve in a conducting medium; record *A* is taken with the electrode touching the

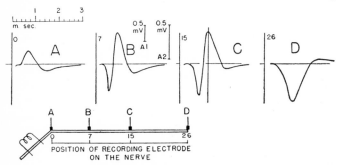

FIG. 37. EFFECT ON THE RECORD OF THE ACTION POTENTIAL OF INCREASING DISTANCE BETWEEN STIMULATING AND RECORDING ELECTRODES

In every case the recording electrode is touching the nerve and the second electrode is on a remote inactive point.
A, the action potential obtained with the recording electrode at the point where the nerve enters the conducting medium; *B*, 7 mm along the nerve; *C*, 15 mm; and *D*, 26 mm along the nerve and at its end. The technique used is described in the text.
(Redrawn from Lorente de Nó (1947) *A Study of Nerve Physiology*. Rockefeller Institute.)

nerve, record *B*, 3 mm from the nerve, and record *C*, 10 mm from the nerve. As the distance between the stimulus and the recording electrode increases (as in Fig. 37), the action spikes broaden and become lower in amplitude; as the electrode moves farther from the surface of the nerve the spikes also lose in amplitude but show rather less broadening (see Fig. 38).

The purpose of this analysis is to point out the influence of extraneural physical factors on the shape and time sequence of the recordings obtained from nerves in their physiological setting, and to emphasise the distinction it is necessary to make between the electrical concomitant of a neuronal process (such as, for example, the positive after-potential) and factors introduced by the recording conditions (such as the positive field created by the departing impulse in a conducting medium). Nerve potential characteristics in a conducting medium are much closer to those occurring in the body than is the behaviour of the isolated nerve in a dielectric medium.

In the central nervous system the lack of homogeneity in volume conductor properties is an added complexity. Neuronal

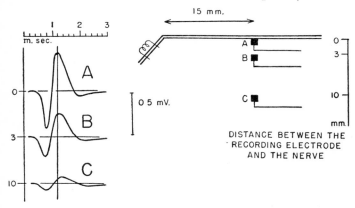

FIG. 38. EFFECT ON THE RECORD OF THE ACTION POTENTIAL OF INCREASING DISTANCE BETWEEN NERVE AND RECORDING ELECTRODE

A, the action potential obtained with the recording electrode touching the nerve; *B*, 3 mm from it; and *C*, 10 mm from it. In every case the second electrode is on a remote inactive point. The technique is described in the text and was similar to that used for establishing Fig. 37.

(Redrawn from Lorente de Nó (1947) *A Study of Nerve Physiology.* Rockefeller Institute.)

tissues have about four or more times the resistivity of normal saline and, since that of white matter is greater than that of grey, distortion of the field results. Even in the spinal cord this causes unequal amplitudes of sources and sinks; when attempts are made to plot the fields in or on convoluted cortex, further distortions are introduced, for part of the field, for example the source, may lie deep and confined in a sulcus while its other part, the sink, spreads out over the surface. Nevertheless, no interpretation of the electrical record can be reached without an understanding of the fundamental characteristics of the simplest case: namely, the spread of electricity in a conducting medium.

BIBLIOGRAPHY

Bishop, G. H. (1937) La théorie des circuits locaux, permet-elle de prévoir la forme du potential d'action? *Arch. int. Physiol.*, **45**, 273.

Bishop, G. H. and O'Leary, J. (1942) Factors determining the form of the potential record in the vicinity of the synapses of the dorsal nucleus of the lateral geniculate body. *J. cell. comp. Physiol.*, **19**, 315.

Brazier, M. A. B. (1949) The electrical fields at the surface of the head during sleep. *Electroenceph. clin. Neurophysiol.*, **1**, 195–204.

Brazier, M. A. B. (1950) The electrical fields at the surface of the head. 2nd Int. EEG Congress. *Electroenceph. clin. Neurophysiol.*, Suppl. 2.

Freeman, W. F. (1963) The electrical activity of a primary sensory cortex: analysis of EEG waves. *Internat. Rev. Biol.*, **5**, 53–119.

Freeman, W. J. (1959) Distribution in time and space of prepyriform electrical activity. *J. Neurophysiol.*, **22**, 644–665.

Freygang, W. H. and Landau, W. M. (1955) Some relations between resistivity and electrical activity in the cerebral cortex of the cat. *J. cell. comp. Physiol.*, **45**, 377–392.

Van Harreveld, A., Hooper, N. K. and Cusick, J. T. (1961) Brain electrolytes and cortical impedance. *Amer. J. Physiol.*, **201**, 139–143.

Von Helmholtz, H. (1853) Über einige Gesetze der Vertheilung elektrischer Ströme in körperlichen Leitern, mit Anwendung auf die thierischelektrischen Versuche. *Ann. Physik. Chem.*, **89**, 211–233 and 353–377.

Lorente de Nó, R. (1947) *A Study of Nerve Physiology*. Rockefeller Institute, New York.

Mauro, A. (1960) Properties of thin generators pertaining to electrophysiological potentials in volume conductors. *J. Neurophysiol.*, **23**, 132–143.

Porter, R., Adey, W. R. and Kado, R. T. (1964) Measurement of electrical impedance in the human brain. *Neurology (Minneap.)*, **14**, 1002–1012.

Ranck, J. B. (1963) Analysis of specific impedance of rabbit cerebral cortex. *Exp. Neurol.*, **7**, 153–174.

Rogers, W. A. (1954) *Introduction to Electric Fields*. McGraw-Hill, New York.

8

The Electrical Excitation of Nerve

In Chapter 6 evidence was presented for a mechanism of propagation of the nerve impulse by local electric currents produced by the nerve itself. Further insight into the physical properties of nerve can therefore be gained by studying the effect of applied currents whose parameters are known. Before techniques for recording from the inside of nerve cells had been developed, all the studies were of peripheral axons subjected to externally applied stimuli and it was from these experiments that the fundamental properties were first established.

When a current of subthreshold intensity and of very short duration is applied to a nerve no action potential is propagated but a disturbance is set up which outlasts for a short time the duration of the pulse. This disturbance set up by an electrical stimulus was named by Keith Lucas the 'local excitatory state' and was thought by him to be a purely local effect, a polarisation at the cathode. In fact the applied current does not merely flow directly through that part of the nerve between the electrodes only (as it would in a wire) but spreads out for a considerable distance along the nerve on either side of the electrodes. Such an effect results from the fact that the nerve behaves like a core conductor separated from a conducting environment by a membrane with some impedance, as Hermann suggested long ago. This longitudinal spread of current is called *electrotonus*; its density falls off exponentially with increasing distance from the electrode, and when the applied current is shut off, the electrotonic potential decays exponentially with time.

A schematic representation of the electrotonic spread along a nerve fibre envisaged as a core conductor is shown in Fig. 39(*b*). This may be compared with Fig. 29 in Chapter 6. That the current spreads in this way is shown by the fact that recording electrodes placed on the nerve beyond the segment which lies

between the stimulating electrodes register a potential difference when a subliminal current is applied to the nerve. This
has been shown for nerve by several workers. The method used
by Lorente de Nó is shown in Fig. 39(a). The stimulating
current is applied through electrodes p_1 and p_2 and the recording
electrodes are at r_1 and r_2. He established that the distance
between the stimulating cathode p_1 and the nearest recording

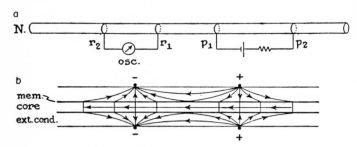

FIG. 39. ELECTROTONUS IN A NERVE FIBRE

(a) Circuit used by Lorente de Nó to demonstrate a potential difference
between electrodes r_1 and r_2 caused by electrotonic spread of the stimulating
current applied at p_1.
(b) Schematic diagram of electrotonic spread in a longitudinal core
conductor separated from the external conducting medium by a membrane
of lower conductivity.
(From Lorente de Nó (1946–7) *Harvey Lect.*, **42**, 43.)

electrode r_1 can be as great as 30–40 mm and still a difference in
potential can be recorded between r_1 and r_2. As the electrode
r_1 is moved away from the cathodal stimulus the recorded
potential difference decays exponentially. The decay of this
potential change with time also shows an approximately
exponential decrement.

The time-lag of decay of the electrotonus has the effect of
lowering the threshold for excitation for a short time so that a
second subthreshold stimulus may evoke a propagated impulse
provided it falls within a certain interval after the first, for the
local change, as we have seen, soon dies away. This critical
interval, the period of *latent addition*, varies in duration for
different tissues. In mammalian A fibres this is about 0·2 msec
in duration but is longer in cold-blooded animals. Unlike the
nerve impulse, electrotonus has no refractory period and it is,
therefore, a different physical process from the action potential.

In addition, it differs from the conducted impulse in being, within limits, proportional to the strength of the stimulus. It does not, therefore, obey the all-or-nothing law.

The effect just described is a summation, a latent addition, not of the action potential or of any conducted process, but of the electrotonus in the fibre surrounding the site of stimulation. The only type of summation of propagated impulses which takes place in single fibres (in contrast with polyneuronal chains) is temporal and is found when the stimuli are so exactly timed that the second falls in the super-normal phase of the recovery period following the first (as described on page 37).

Another effect is seen in the nerve at the point of stimulation when the current is shut off. This results in a fall of excitability, not only to the resting baseline but below it. This is known as postcathodal depression (see below, page 87).

Clearly, if the initiation of a propagated impulse depends on the building up of a threshold excitatory state, and if the accumulation of this in its turn is proportional to the stimulus, certain factors will be decisive: one is the strength of the stimulating current, and another the duration of its flow. There are, however, lower limits for each of these factors, a duration threshold and an intensity threshold. Rushton found that there is a third factor, that of minimal length: a finite minimal length of nerve has to be excited before a propagated disturbance can be evoked. The minimal current strength below which no propagated response can be elicited, however long the application, is known as the rheobase. The minimum duration for a rheobasic current to be effective is called the utilisation time, or 'temps utile'; unless the current persists at least until the action spike develops, no impulse will result. If a graph is drawn (as in Fig. 40), plotting the duration of the applied stimulus against the threshold intensity necessary to produce an action potential, the rheobase is that point at which the curve flattens out and becomes horizontal, for below this level increasing the duration will be ineffective in producing a response. Such charts are known as strength–duration curves.

The product they depict is related to many of the factors already discussed; one, for example, is conduction velocity; as has been seen, the more rapidly a fibre conducts, the greater its excitability and, therefore, the weaker the current needed to stimulate it. And since fibre size is related to velocity this too will be concerned in the strength–duration curves.

Nernst suggested an explanation of the excitation-time of nerve based on a theory that an electric current draws ions to the membrane against the tendency for diffusion to pull them away. This concentration accumulates with the square root of time ($\sqrt{t}$) and an impulse will be evoked only when the product of the strength of the current and the square root of its duration ($i \times \sqrt{t}$) exceeds a certain threshold value. Nernst's theory

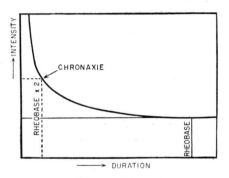

FIG. 40. STRENGTH–DURATION CURVE

holds only within certain limits and many modifications have been suggested, among them Lapique's, that the initiation of an impulse depends not on the actual concentration of ions at the point of stimulation but on the concentration gradient across the membrane. Another modification was formerly advanced by Hill who stressed the semipermeable nature of the membrane and suggested that the accommodation to a constant current was a rise in the threshold of the nerve evoked by the stimulus (see page 86). This would be comparable to an early cathodal depression. None of these theories has completely satisfied its author or covered all the observed data.

A derivative of strength–duration curves which has occupied considerable space in neurophysiological texts during the last fifty years is that of *chronaxie*. It is also a subject on which opinion has modified as knowledge has grown. Chronaxie was a term introduced by Lapique to designate the time factor in excitation of tissues including nerves and nerve cells when they are stimulated by a constant current. Lapique defined chron-axie as the least duration of a current which will excite at a strength of double the rheobase and it is, therefore, identical by definition with the 'excitation time' of Keith Lucas. The concept was introduced to fill the need for an index of excitability not only in nerve but in other tissues. It has proved in critical work to be only a rough measure of the time factor in excitation and to be subject to variations contributed by many extraneous factors as has been demonstrated by Forbes, Rushton, and others.

As we have seen, the excitability of fibres is related to conduction velocity—the faster the conduction the greater the excitability, and if chronaxie is to be considered a reliable index of excitability the same relationship with velocity should hold. It has been demonstrated by several workers that there is no direct correlation between chronaxie and conduction velocity. Nor can Lapique's conclusion that the chronaxie of a neurone is uniform throughout all its ramifications be maintained, as it is irreconcilable with the relationship proved to exist between the diameter of the fibre and its conduction rate. Lapique's theory of isochronism which postulates the same excitation time for all components of a motor unit (the nerve, the neuro-muscular junction and the muscle fibre) has also received some criticism and little support from other laboratories. Keith Lucas's demonstration in 1906 of three different chronaxies for nerve, muscle and neuromuscular junction in the toad was in direct opposition to Lapique's theory. Furthermore it has been frequently demonstrated, as Rushton has emphasised, that the value obtained for chronaxie depends on the type of electrodes used, the larger the electrode the longer the excitation time. Clearly chronaxie cannot be regarded as characteristic of the tissue alone. For these reasons, among others, chronaxie is not generally held to be a satisfactory index of excitability of nerve.

The discussion so far has been on the effect of the switching on of a monophasic current (a rectangular pulse) which has the effect of exciting at the cathode. This causes a depolarisa-tion of the membrane, i.e. a decrease in negativity inside the membrane at the cathode and the region surrounding it (cate-lectrotonus), and a simultaneous increase in internal positivity at the anodal region (anelectrotonus). On the break of the current, this positive charge at the anode collapses and the membrane potential at that region returns to its resting level. This local reversal of charge is equivalent to a depolarisation and accounts for the excitation at the anode on the break of the current. Especially in the central nervous system and in experiments *in vivo*, care is taken to avoid the duration of de-polarisation being long enough to cause injury. A form of stimulus which has proved generally satisfactory is a diphasic rectangular pulse, each phase of which has a duration no longer than 1/10 msec.

If the constant current is not broken but allowed to flow continuously, the nerve usually does not continue to respond. The question has been raised by Bishop as to whether this may not be a laboratory artefact consequent to some injury having been done to the nerve. Certainly some invertebrate nerves can be induced to respond repetitively to stimulation by a constant current, as is described later in Chapter 11 (see also Fig. 70). A related effect is found with a very slowly increasing stimulus, where, except with currents of great strength, a gradual increase of intensity fails to evoke a response in the nerve. This effect was named by Nernst 'Akkommodation'. In the German language such gradually-rising stimuli are graphically described as 'einschleichende' or creeping. In both these situations the quality of rapid change is missing from the stimulus, and it is exactly this property which is required to evoke persistent activity in the fibre. The nerve is still excitable, but it needs what Keith Lucas described as a 'minimal gradient' of stimula-tion. Since this early formulation, more modern techniques have shown this to be true for the single nerve fibre and the single Ranvier node.

The time factors involved in these two phenomena, the decay of the local excitatory process during the passage of a constant current, and the change of threshold to slowly increasing cur-rents, called 'accommodation', were the subject of extensive studies by Solandt and by Hill and his co-workers who regard the nerve fibre as behaving like a leaky condenser. The time factor for accommodation is always the larger of the two and has been measured for many types of nerve. In human ulnar nerve this time constant is approximately 60 msec.

The fibres of sensory nerves have far less accommodation than those of motor nerves, and the fine pain fibres have almost none. This is illustrated in Fig. 41 (taken from Skoglund's studies), in which the rate of four linearly-rising currents is graphically represented by the four fine lines fanning out from zero. A circle is plotted at the point where each of these rising currents produces a threshold response from the nerve. The line joining

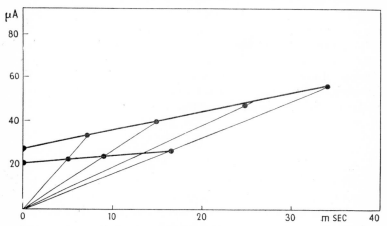

FIG. 41. ACCOMMODATION CURVES FOR MOTOR AND SENSORY NERVE
Upper thick line: motor nerve. Lower thick line: sensory nerve. Fine lines represent the rate of four linearly-increasing currents from which the plots were made.
(From Skoglund (1942) *Acta physiol. scand.*, **4**, Supplement 12.)

all these points is the accommodation curve for the nerve. The initial point plotted on the ordinate at the zero value of the abscissa is the rheobase at which a constant current just evokes a response. The upper thick line is the accommodation curve of a motor nerve, the lower thick line is that of a sensory nerve. The former shows more accommodation, as is indicated by the steeper slope.

Mathematical equations descriptive of the behaviour of nerves on stimulation by constant currents have been proposed by Monnier, by Rashevsky and by Hill, and their respective theories have been critically examined by Lefevre. A simple expression suggested by Hill for the decay (with a constant stimulus) of the local excitatory state or local potential from its level V, when initially stimulated, down to the baseline potential V_0 of the resting state is as follows—

$$- \frac{dV}{dt} = (V - V_0) \, K$$

According to this formula the rate of fall in potential is a direct function of the difference between the initial and the final potential values, K being the time-constant of excitation, i.e. the rate of decay of the excitatory state.

The other time factor, which is quite independent, is the time-constant of accommodation, a measure of the rate of change of current strength necessary to achieve the threshold for excitation; it has been calculated by Hill and may be expressed in its simplest form as follows—

$$\frac{dV}{dt} = \frac{(U - U_0)}{\lambda}$$

Or expressed in words, 'the rate of change of local potential (V) is related to the difference between the threshold (U_0) at which a rapidly applied stimulus of adequate strength excites, and the final raised threshold (U) at which the slowly-rising current at last evokes an impulse'. The constant, λ, is the time-constant of accommodation, and is, therefore, a measure of the rate of change of the threshold of excitation. If this rate of change of threshold is slower than the rate of rise of local potential the nerve will continue to discharge; if $\dfrac{dV}{dt}$ is slower than $\dfrac{dU}{dt}$ the discharge will cease.

Attempts have been made to suggest theories of excitation which would be susceptible to mathematical formulation. One of these, advanced by Lapique and developed by Blair, was that when a current is applied the dimensions of a single process are responsible for excitation in nerve. Rashevsky has suggested a modification of the theory very similar to that of Hill in which he conceives of a balance between two antagonistic factors, e and i (a rapid excitatory, and a slow inhibitory process), each varying with the current. Only when e/i reaches a critical threshold value does excitation result.

Interpreted according to the membrane hypothesis, excitation occurs when the rate of concentration of the excitatory ions exceeds the rate of restoration of the resting equilibrium. According to Lorente de Nó's views both adaptation and accommodation are due to a reaction of the nerve, in opposition to the applied current, tending to re-establish equilibrium: there is an increase of the e.m.f. of the membrane if the stimulus is cathodal and a decrease in the e.m.f. if it is anodal. The nerve always reacts to the applied stimulus and never behaves like a passive structure. This is the familiar phenomenon of polarisation where a back e.m.f. is built up in opposition to the imposed current. The opposing e.m.f. of the membrane is revealed when the applied cathodal current is suddenly shut off, for the nerve reaction lags and an overshooting of its potential appears as a positive deflection in the record. In physiological terms this would seem to be a marshalling of metabolic mechanisms in the nerve to replace the charged particles that are removed from the double layers by the imposed current. This is the post-cathodal depression mentioned above. The opposite effect takes place under the anode where, at the end of the stimulating current, there is a short period of enhanced excitability. In a nerve already made highly excitable by citration (that is, by inactivation of the Ca ion) this postanodal enhancement can be made to oscillate and if the negative swing becomes great enough a propagated action potential may result. This phenomenon has received intensive study from Monnier, from Fessard, and from Arvanitaki.

The observation has been made by Hodgkin and by Katz that as a result of a just subthreshold electrical stimulus there is not only an electrotonic potential but also a response due to the nerve itself producing an additional negativity under the cathode. With subliminal stimuli this response is spatially too limited to initiate a propagated action potential. Hodgkin suggested that the condition for excitation was that the cathodic response must reach a potential at which it can propagate through the nerve by local circuit action. He called this active stationary process the 'local response' and framed this hypothesis as an interpretation of his findings in single (unmyelinated) fibres of crustacean nerve. Katz's finding of local responses in frog's myelinated nerve supports Hodgkin's hypothesis, as does later work by Rosenblueth.

Lorente de Nó has made the proposition that the reaction of

the nerve to the impressed current by the building-up of an opposing e.m.f. in the membrane may itself be the initiator of the nerve impulse. This building-up of the back e.m.f. proceeds as long as it is insufficient to excite the fibre. When it reaches the threshold for excitation the nerve suddenly and rapidly

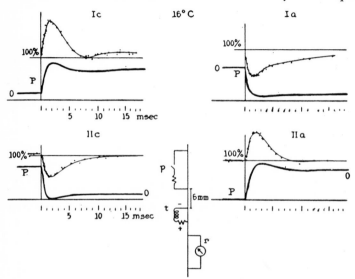

FIG. 42. COMPARISON OF ELECTROTONIC POTENTIALS AND EXCITABILITY IN NERVE FIBRES

The heavier line P of each pair of curves represents the electrotonic potential, the finer line, the excitability (frog nerve). Ic is at the make, IIc after the break of a cathodal current. Ia is at the make, IIa after the break of an anodal current.

(From Lorente de Nó (1946–7) *Harvey Lect.*, **42,** 43.)

depolarises, thus initiating the impulse. In support of the evidence for this hypothesis is his demonstration of the close parallelism between the amplitude of this opposing e.m.f. and the excitability curve of the nerve. In Fig. 42 the comparison is made between the electrotonic potential (shown in the lower curve, P, of each pair) and the excitability (in the upper curve of each pair). Sections Ic and IIc present the changes at the make, and after the break of a cathodal current; Ia and IIa the changes at the make, and after the break of an anodal current. This record also demonstrates the almost exactly similar effect of the make of a cathodal current and the break of an anodal current (and vice versa), an observation originally made by Pflüger. These studies were made on frog nerve and the time characteristics are consequently slower than for mammalian nerve.

Many equivalent circuits have been proposed from time to time, each illustrative of the proponent's hypothesis. Reproduced in Fig. 43 is the one proposed by Hodgkin and Huxley

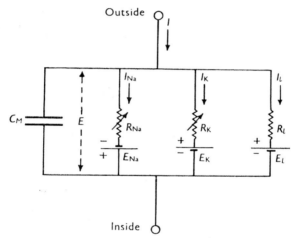

FIG. 43. THE EQUIVALENT CIRCUIT PROPOSED BY HODGKIN AND HUXLEY FOR THE AXON MEMBRANE (SQUID)

Electrical circuit representing membrane. $R_{Na} = 1/g_{Na}$; $R_K = 1/g_K$; $R_l = 1/\bar{g}_l$. R_{Na} and R_K vary with time and membrane potential; the other components are constant.

(From Hodgkin and Huxley, J. (1952) *J. Physiol.* (*Lond.*), **117**, 501.)

in relation to their 'sodium' theory of the action potential (as described in Chapter 6). When the nerve is at rest, the conductance of the membrane is maintained by the permeability of the membrane to potassium ions (g_K). At the peak of activity g_{Na} increases and exceeds g_K, and the membrane potential reverses from its resting level (E_K) to the new level E_{Na}.

Most of the studies of electrical excitation of nerve have been by direct currents. When an alternating current is used it is found that there is an optimal frequency for excitation—below this frequency the gradient of increasing strength of current is too gentle to excite, and above the optimal frequency the duration of each impulse becomes too short. The most favourable frequency for excitation of mammalian nerve by an alternating current is approximately 100 c/s.

BIBLIOGRAPHY

Adrian, E. D. and Lucas, K. (1912) On the summation of propagated disturbances in nerve and muscle. *J. Physiol. (Lond.)*, **44**, 68–124.

Arvanitaki, A. (1939) 'Les variations graduées de la polarisation des systèmes excitables.' In *Physiologie Générale du Système Nerveux.* Hermann, Paris.

Bishop, G. H. (1928) The effect of nerve reactance on the threshold of nerve during galvanic current flow. *Amer. J. Physiol.*, **84**, 417–436.

Bishop, G. H. (1951) 'Excitability.' In *The Nerve Impulse.* No. 2. Josiah Macy Jr. Foundation.

Blair, H. A. (1936) The kinetics of the excitatory process. *Cold Spr. Harb. Symp. quant. Biol.*, **4**, 63–72.

Cole, K. S. (1962) The advance of electrical models for cells and axons. *Biophys. J.*, **2**, Suppl., 101–119.

Conway, B. E. (1965) *Theory and Principles of Electrode Processes.* Ronald Press, New York.

Davis, H. and Forbes, A. (1936) Chronaxie. *Physiol. Rev.*, **16**, 407–441.

Fessard, A. (1936) *Recherches sur l'activité rhythmique des nerfs isolés.* Hermann, Paris.

Franck, U. F. (1956) Models for biological excitation phenomena. *Progr. Biophys.*, **6**, 171–206.

Hill, A. V. (1936) Excitation and accommodation in nerve. *Proc. roy. Soc. B.*, **119**, 305–355.

Hill, A. V. (1936) The strength-duration relation for electric excitation of medullated nerve. *Proc. roy. Soc. B.*, **119**, 440–453.

Hodgkin, A. L. (1938) The subthreshold potentials in a crustacean nerve fibre. *Proc. roy. Soc. B.*, **126**, 87–121.

Hodgkin, A. L. and Rushton, W. A. H. (1946) The electrical constants of a crustacean nerve fibre. *Proc. roy. Soc. B.*, **133**, 444–479.

Hodgkin, A. L. and Huxley, A. F. (1952) A quantitative description of membrane current and its application to conduction and excitation in nerve. *J. Physiol.*, **117**, 500–544.

Katz, B. (1939) *Electric Excitation of Nerve.* Oxford University Press, London.

Katz, B. (1947) Subthreshold potentials in medullated nerve. *J. Physiol.*, **106**, 66–79.

Katz, B. (1966) *Nerve, Muscle, and Synapse*. McGraw-Hill Book Company, New York.

Kugelberg, E. (1944) Accommodation in human nerves. *Acta physiol. scand.*, **8**, Suppl. 24.

Lapique, L. (1926) *L'Excitabilité en Fonction du Temps*. Hermann, Paris.

LeFevre, P. G. (1950) Excitation characteristics in giant squid axon. A test of excitation theory in a case of rapid accommodation. *J. gen. Physiol.*, **34**, 19–36.

Lorente de Nó, R. (1947) Correlation of nerve activity with polarisation phenomena. *Harvey Lect.*, **42**, 43–105.

Lucas, K. (1907) On the rate of variation of the exciting current as a factor in electric excitation. *J. Physiol. (Lond.)*, **36**, 253–274.

Monnier, A. M. (1934) *L'Excitation Électrique des Tissus*. Hermann, Paris.

Monnier, A. M. (1952) The damping factor as a functional criterion in nerve physiology. *Cold Spr. Harb. Symp. quant. Biol.*, **17**, 69–92.

Nernst, W. (1908) Zur Theorie des electrischen Reizes. *Pflügers. Arch. ges. Physiol.*, **122**, 275–314.

Rashevsky, N. (1960) *Mathematical Biophysics*. Dover Publications, New York.

Rosenblueth, A. and Luco, J. V. (1950) The local responses of myelinated mammalian axons. *J. cell. comp. Physiol.*, **36**, 289–331.

Rushton, W. A. H. (1927) The effect upon the threshold for nervous excitation of the length of nerve exposed and the angle between current and nerve. *J. Physiol. (Lond.)*, **63**, 357–377.

Rushton, W. A. H. (1935) The time factor in electrical excitation. *Biol. Rev.*, **10**, 1.

Skoglund, C. G. (1942) The response to linearly increasing currents in mammalian motor and sensory nerves. *Acta physiol. scand.*, **4**, Suppl., 12.

Solandt, D. Y. (1936) The measurement of accommodation. *Proc. roy. Soc. B.*, **119**, 355–379.

Tasaki, I. (1953) *Nervous Transmission*. Thomas, Springfield.

9

Transmission at Synapses and at the Neuromuscular Junction

As mentioned in Chapter 1, transmission of impulses between nerve cells is apparently across a junction, for in vertebrates there is no known continuity of nervous tissue from one neurone to another. The junction was called by Sherrington the *synapse*, and the complex patterns of its function in the nervous system are decisive in the integration of nervous action.

An outstanding property of a synapse is that transmission across it is essentially in one direction only. Another characteristic of the synapse is that it causes a delay in a message, for it takes time for impulses in presynaptic fibres to initiate another impulse in a neurone across a synapse. Forbes and his co-workers found the synaptic delay in the flexion reflex in the cat to be about 3 msec for the first stimulus, but after repeated stimulation the synaptic time was reduced to about 0·6 msec or less.

These figures were calculated from recordings made from the whole nerve with extracellular electrodes, but were found to be surprisingly accurate when checked by the modern techniques of intracellular recordings; these can determine more precisely the exact onset of the postsynaptic potential, though not of the arrival time of the presynaptic potential, since the nerve terminals are too fine to admit the inserted electrode very close to the ending. In general the lower figures for transmission at central and neuromuscular synapses were confirmed (0·3 msec or slightly less for mammalian synapses). In the autonomic system and in the invertebrate synapses, the delay is much longer.

Another important characteristic of synaptic transmission is that the end-fibres of many axons impinge on the same secondary neurone; also, the profusely branching end-fibres of one neurone may make synaptic connexion with many others. It is unlikely that the simple case of a single fibre synapsing with a single secondary neurone ever occurs in the human nervous

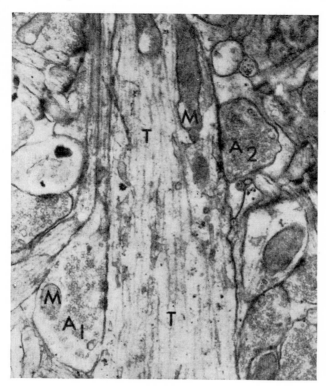

FIG. 44. AXO-DENDRITIC SYNAPSES

Electron micrograph of a large dendrite (*T*) seen longitudinally. Two axons (*A*₁ and *A*₂) form synapses on this dendrite, *A*₁ being cut longitudinally so that its long, narrow preterminal process is clearly seen. *M* = mitochondria. Thalamus of the cat.

(By courtesy of Dr. George Pappas.)

system. Each cell lies in a forest of arborising fibre-endings and these presynaptic terminals may make connexion with the cell body, its dendrites or its axon. Such synapses are known as axo-somatic, axo-dendritic and axo-axonal respectively (see Fig. 44).

As just mentioned, many presynaptic endings may make

synaptic contact with the same postsynaptic neurone. When these multiple presynaptic fibres are activated simultaneously, the amplitude of the resulting postsynaptic potential is a simple summation of the individual ones. Spatial summation is, therefore, a marked characteristic of these graded responses.

A mass effect of summation is seen in the phenomenon of *facilitation*. This name is given to the situation in which a series of impulses may induce in a neuronal field a state of subliminal excitation—insufficient alone to propagate impulses in the postsynaptic neurones. Only with the added effect of further impulses entering along other axons and impinging on the same neuronal field is transmission of messages across these synapses effected. The latter set of impulses is said to be facilitated by the pre-established state of subliminal excitability.

In spinal reflexes, successive stimuli to many neighbouring receptors may enhance the response in the final common path. This is well illustrated by the scratch reflex of the dog. A gentle touch, too weak to effect a motor response, may, if drawn along the skin, elicit the reflex result: the dog scratches his skin. Sherrington suggested that it may be the hop of the flea that has saved this species from extinction, as in this way it avoids recruiting successive spatially separate stimuli and resultant annihilation by the scratching foot.

It was effects of this nature that Sherrington called the *central excitatory state*, and in addition he postulated a corollary, *the central inhibitory state*. At the time when he was developing these hypotheses, techniques for recording from single neurones had not been developed and Sherrington's formulation was necessarily rather a global one, though it is of interest to note that as long ago as 1932 Sherrington suggested that 'the inhibitory stabilisation of the membrane might be pictured as a heightening of the "resting" polarisation . . .' As will be seen from the section below on transmission of impulses to single neurones (page 102), more detailed information is now available from which to frame a hypothesis as to the neural events responsible for the observed facts.

Sherrington described the central excitatory state as a long-persisting, slowly-decaying phase of high excitability that could be added to by the arrival of any subsequent impulses. His concept therefore covered, among other phenomena, many of the effects now known to be due to varying numbers of inter-neurones lying in the path of excitation.

Forbes, in 1921, demonstrated the importance in the reflex of the convergence of many afferent conducting paths, or their central connexions, at a single motor neurone and pointed out that a varying number of interneurones in these paths would result in an enduring response such as has just been described.

Facilitation of impulses by the very recent setting up of a field of short-lasting subliminal excitation was thought for a long time to be the only form of this activity, but in the '30s several schemata were suggested for activity in closed circuits of neurones which could serve as self re-exciting chains. Impulses circulating in such loops would have a facilitating influence on all impulses arriving along axons synaptically related to any of their constituent neurones. Two of the first schemata to be proposed are illustrated. On the left of Fig. 45 is Ranson's sketch of a network to account for the after-discharges in hind-limb reflexes, and on the right Lorente de Nó's schema for a self re-exciting chain of neurones in the oculomotor nucleus. These early conceptual formulations have led to many of the mathematical models being proposed today for simulation of neuronal networks.

The presence of recurrent neuronal pathways has now been demonstrated in several phyla and the possible roles of these structures are being investigated in many laboratories. Since the energy for all nerve impulses comes from the fibres them-selves, activity in such structures could circulate almost indefi-nitely provided the metabolism of the constituent neurones were maintained; in this way a long persisting effect set up by an initial stimulus would serve to facilitate impulses coming later in the life of the organism. This type of integration in the central nervous system has been suggested as a neuronal basis for one form of learning and short-term memory. Supportive experimental evidence for the role that self re-exciting neuronal loops may play in the learning process may be found in the work of Young on cuttlefish. Learned responses in these animals are 'forgotten' if specific circular nerve tracts are sectioned.

Transmission through sympathetic ganglia has been studied extensively. Incoming impulses have been recorded in the preganglionic fibres and traced through to the fibres on the other side of the ganglionic synapses. A typical record of an action potential produced by stimulation of the preganglionic nerve trunk is reproduced in Fig. 46. With one electrode on the ganglion and the other on the postganglionic nerve the initial

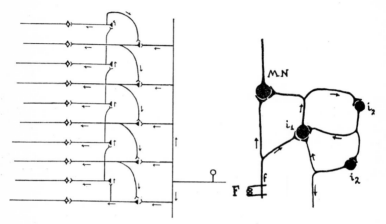

FIG. 45. TWO SUGGESTED SCHEMATA FOR REVERBERATING NEURONE CIRCUITS

Left: A single volley from the nerve cell on the right would produce, in the series of motor neurones on the left, a long-lasting asynchronous shower of discharges. This circuit could account for extensor after-discharges lasting many seconds in hind limb reflexes.

(From Ranson and Hinsey (1930) *Amer. J. Physiol.*, **94,** 471.)

Right: A schema for a self re-exciting chain of neurones in the oculomotor nucleus. A stimulus to fibre *F* might be subliminal alone for stimulation of motor neurone *MN*, but would create a rhythmic series of impulses in the circular pathways through the network of neurones, so that the subsequent impulses from the fibre *F* could be facilitated by the activity in neurone i_1.

(From Lorente de Nó (1935) *Amer. J. Physiol.*, **113,** 505.)

response is a spike potential in which the ganglion cells are briefly strongly negative to their axons. This is followed by another slower negative potential during which the threshold of excitation is lowered, and later by a long-lasting positive surge during which the threshold is raised.

These classic studies of transmission in sympathetic ganglia were made by Eccles before intracellular techniques were developed. Twenty years and a generation later, postganglionic potentials were recorded from inside mammalian sympathetic ganglia. In the upper section of Fig. 46, is Eccles's original picture of the postsynaptic potential recorded extracellularly from a sympathetic ganglion in the cat, and below is the intra-cellular record of R. M. Eccles taken from the superior cervical

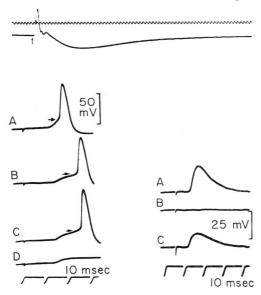

FIG. 46. ACTION POTENTIAL OF A GANGLION CELL

Above: Response to a single induction shock to the presynaptic trunk of a sympathetic ganglion in the cat. Time signal: 10 msec.

(From Eccles (1935) *J. Physiol. (Lond.),* **85,** 176.)

Below: On the left, action potentials recorded intracellularly from the superior cervical ganglion of a rabbit in response to a single presynaptic volley decreasing in stimulus strength from *A* to *D.* On the right, two examples of postsynaptic potentials that did not reach threshold for spike discharge in *A* or *C.* In *B* the stimulus was too weak to evoke an EPSP.

(From Eccles (1955) *J. Physiol. (Lond.),* **130,** 572.)

ganglion of a rabbit. In both cases the action potential was evoked by a presynaptic shock.

The intracellular records show very clearly that the post-ganglionic spike arises from a postsynaptic potential, provided the latter reaches the threshold for discharge. Since the post-synaptic potential is a graded one whose amplitude can sum, the greater the intensity of the presynaptic volley, the sooner the threshold for discharge is reached and, therefore, the latency to the spike is an index of intensity of the stimulus.

Larrabee and Bronk have found that sympathetic ganglion cells continue to discharge rhythmic impulses for many seconds after the end of a brief repetitive stimulation of the preganglionic nerve. Although the frequency of stimulation needs to be higher than would be found physiologically, this after-discharge is of particular interest since sympathetic ganglia certainly contain no interneurones and they therefore furnish an example of one type of prolonged excitatory state which cannot be due to activity in chains of interneurones.

It is, of course, an oversimplification to speak of the preganglionic fibre of a sympathetic ganglion cell. Many fibres converge on each ganglion cell and therefore discharges of different frequencies may be reaching the cell simultaneously. In addition, the terminal branches of any one presynaptic fibre may tangle with many ganglion cells. Eccles has recognised in this multiple innervation of ganglion cells the situation originally described by Sherrington for spinal reflexes: that of occlusion. The fact that several postsynaptic neurones share innervation results in a reduction of response if the presynaptic fibres are fired synchronously instead of consecutively. It is this reduction of response which is termed *occlusion*. It is illustrated by Sherrington's well-known diagram reproduced in Fig. 47.

In this diagram presynaptic fibre a is seen to innervate four postsynaptic neurones, and of these four, two are also innervated by presynaptic fibre b. Adequate stimulation of fibre a alone will activate four postsynaptic fibres: α', α, α'', and β'. Adequate stimulation of fibre b will also activate four postsynaptic fibres: β', β, β'', and α'. However, strong simultaneous stimulation of a and b will result in activation, not of eight postsynaptic neurones, but of six. Neurones α' and β' are shared by occlusion. Facilitation is shown diagrammatically in a similar way. Impulses coming into the neuronal pool will not only directly activate certain neurones (α and β in diagram B) but will also have a subliminal excitatory effect on neighbouring nerve cells (the spatial spread of electrotonus similar to that already referred to on page 64). If any of these subliminally excited cells lie also within reach of the electrotonus evoked by a discharge from another presynaptic fibre, summation may

occur and result in a transmitted impulse. This is illustrated
in section B of Sherrington's figure (Fig. 47), where the areas
of the pool influenced by eddy currents (the subliminal fringe)
are enclosed in broken lines.   Postsynaptic neurones α' and β'
in this diagram lie in the electrotonic field common to activity
in both presynaptic fibres. They discharge by facilitation due
to spatial summation. This is not the same type of facilitation
as that due to the *temporal summation* of two impulses in the same

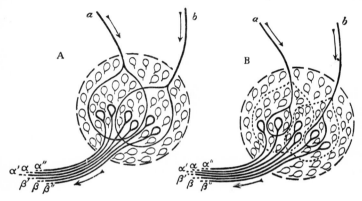

FIG. 47.

Sherrington's classic diagrams to illustrate: *A*, Occlusion; *B*, Facilitation
in a pool of neurones. (For explanation see text.)
(From Sherrington (1929) *Proc. roy. Soc. B.*, **105,** 332.)

fibre, the second of which reaches the cell during the supernormal period of the negative after-potential, i.e. the period of
post-spike residual depolarisation, caused by the first action
potential (see page 37).
    The ultimate response in the postganglionic nerve trunk is
determined by the frequency of impulses arriving at each
synapse and the number of synapses at which they arrive. Even
subliminal impulses will ultimately affect the outcome if they
persist long enough, for they will eventually summate provided
the time relations are suitable. The longer the stimulation lasts,
the more ganglion cells are then recruited. Since the postganglionic nerve follows the frequency of a rhythmic electrical
stimulation applied to the preganglionic nerve, this *recruitment*
can be very clearly demonstrated. In Fig. 48, taken from Bronk,

a rhythmic sequence of shocks of uniform strength was given to the preganglionic nerve trunk; the record is of the action spikes in the postganglionic trunk and shows clearly by the rising height of the spike the progressive recruitment of ganglion cells.

The stimulation of preganglionic fibres frees acetylcholine and potassium in the sympathetic ganglion; both of these substances increase the excitability of the cell body, in contrast to calcium which depresses it. Conduction across the synapse in the sympathetic ganglion is, however, as resistant to asphyxia as in the fibres, although the synapses of the central nervous

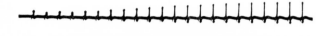

FIG. 48. PROGRESSIVE RECRUITMENT OF GANGLION CELLS DURING RHYTHMIC STIMULATION OF THE PREGANGLIONIC NERVE TRUNK

The record shows the action spikes from the postganglionic nerve. Time signal: 0·5 msec.

(From Bronk (1939) *J. Neurophysiol.*, **2**, 380.)

system seem quite vulnerable to asphyxia. These facts are part of the basis for the chemical theory of synaptic conduction in which the inference is made that acetylcholine is the synaptic transmitter in ganglia.

The sympathetic ganglion with its single preganglionic nerve trunk is more easily studied than the synapses of the central nervous system, for activation of this single trunk is the sole route to the ganglion, and the postganglionic trunk is the sole egress from it. In the central nervous system the connexions are far more complex since fibres from many different nerve trunks synapse with the same neurones and each nerve trunk may synapse to several final paths. It follows that impulses in one fibre, since it connects with so many cells, may facilitate the effect of impulses in other neurones and the conditions for response in any given cell group are a complex of these effects.

SYNAPTIC TRANSMISSION TO SINGLE CELLS

Current knowledge of the behaviour of single neurones results from the development of intracellular recording. First developed by Brock, Coombs and Eccles for the large motor neurones in the mammalian spinal cord, this has since been achieved by many investigators in less massive cells including those of the neocortex. The relative sizes of the anterior horn cell and of the microelectrode used by the pioneer workers is shown in Fig. 49.

For many years the mechanism of conduction of nerve impulses across synapses was a matter of controversy, hypotheses of electrical transmission and of chemical transmission both

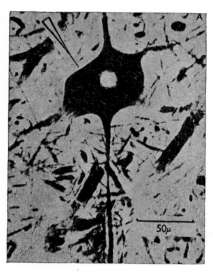

FIG. 49. PHOTOMICROGRAPH OF A MOTOR NEURONE FROM A CAT'S SPINAL CORD SHOWING THE CELL BODY WITH DENDRITES, THE AXON HILLOCK, AND THE AXON RUNNING DOWN TO THE BOTTOM OF THE PICTURE

Superimposed is a sketch of the microelectrode tip, drawn to scale in order to demonstrate relative sizes.

(From Brock, Coombs and Eccles (1952) *J. Physiol. (Lond.)*, **117,** 431.)

having had their proponents. In the last few years, however, incontrovertible evidence has accumulated in support of the chemical theory. The latter states that all synaptic transmission in the vertebrates is chemically mediated. This means, in effect, that a nerve impulse travelling down an axon (by electrical propagation) on reaching the axon terminals has a secretory effect that releases there a chemical transmitter. It is this chemical mediation that affects the receptor membrane of the postsynaptic membrane. There is certainly more than one chemical transmitter and these may have different actions. Some (the excitors) depolarise the postjunctional membrane making a local area of low threshold. In other words, there is a reduction in the potential difference between the inside and the outside of the recipient neurone. This is a non-propagated local response, an electrotonic potential that falls off exponentially with increasing distance from the junctional point. This

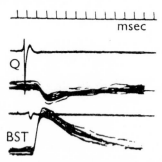

FIG. 50. INTRACELLULAR RECORDINGS OF HYPERPOLARISATION DURING INHIBITION, AND DEPOLARISATION DURING EXCITATION

In the record marked Q, the superimposed sweeps show the response of a biceps-semitendinosus motor neurone to stimulation of the Group $1a$ afferents of the monosynaptic pathway to its antagonist muscle (the quadriceps). The downward deflection indicates hyperpolarisation (and inhibition).
In the record marked BST the response of the same cell to stimulation of its own monosynaptic arc is a depolarisation indicative of heightened excitability. (Above each of the multiple sweeps is the afferent volley recorded from the stimulated L6 dorsal root, negativity downwards. Only the last represents a propagated potential change.)
(From Coombs, Eccles and Fatt (1955) *J. Physiol. (Lond.)*, **130,** 396.)

is called the *excitatory postsynaptic potential*, or EPSP for short. There is now evidence that another class of chemical transmitters (the inhibitors) may cause an increase of the negative potential difference across the membrane of the cell, a hyperpolarisation of the postjunctional membrane that prevents the neurone firing. This is called the *inhibitory postsynaptic potential* or IPSP.

The outstanding characteristic of the postsynaptic potential evoked by neuronal activity in the presynaptic fibre is that (unlike the all-or-nothing spike potential that propagates from one part of a neurone to another part) it is a local graded response.

In the excitatory transmitters, the stronger the stimulus (i.e. the greater the number of active presynaptic fibres impinging on a neurone), the greater the degree of depolarisation of the

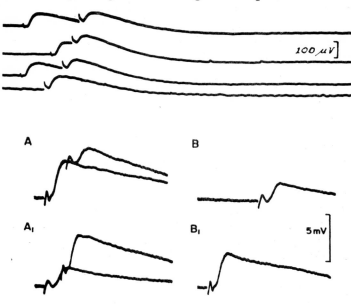

FIG. 51. POSTSYNAPTIC POTENTIALS EVOKED IN A VENTRAL ROOT
BY STIMULI TO THE CORRESPONDING DORSAL ROOT

Above: The lowest record gives the response to a single shock, the other three the summating effect of paired stimuli with different inter-shock intervals.

(From Eccles (1946) *J. Neurophysiol.*, **9**, 87.)

Below: Single cell recordings showing summation of amplitude of excitatory postsynaptic potentials in a single motor neurone of the frog when two different presynaptic fibres are stimulated. In *A*, the lateral column of the spinal cord was stimulated and then the dorsal root. In A_1, the sequence was reversed. In *B* is shown the EPSP evoked by dorsal root stimulation alone and in B_1 of lateral stimulation alone.

(From Fadiga and Brookhart (1962) *J. Neurophysiol.*, **25**, 790.)

membrane across the synapse. The hyperpolarisation effects of the inhibitory transmitters are similarly proportional to the strength of the stimulus.

As a consequence, another characteristic of postsynaptic potentials is that they have no refractory period (see Fig. 51).

Hence, if the synapse receives further neural stimulation, with the release of more transmitter substance before the local response set up by previous stimuli has subsided, the subsequent potential change will add to the pre-existing one.

Summation of postsynaptic potentials can result from either the sequential arrival of impulses in the same presynaptic fibre or from the simultaneous or near simultaneous impingement on to the postsynaptic cell of impulses from more than one presynaptic fibre (as shown in Fig. 51). The transmitter sets up a type of electrogenesis in the postsynaptic membrane that can summate until the degree of depolarisation reaches the critical level for another type of electrogenesis, i.e. the sudden production of an action spike which can then be propagated throughout the length of the postsynaptic neurones in the all-or-nothing, decrementless fashion that has been described in Chapter 6. This is the message carrier to distant parts (see Fig. 52).

Thus, these two types of electrogenesis are quite distinct although they take place in the same neurone. They may be defined as follows: (1) the chemically mediated, trans-synaptically evoked graded response that remains a local response, decrements with increasing distance from the synaptic junction where it originates, and does not make the membrane refractory —hence, additional potentials can sum with it. If this summated effect reaches a certain critical level of depolarisation at the postsynaptic junction (10 mV in spinal motor neurones) it triggers electrogenesis of the second type, namely: (2) the electrically-propagated all-or-nothing decrementless action spike travelling from one part of a neurone to another part of the same neurone leaving a period of refractoriness behind it, and mediated by the influence of membrane breakdown and sodium ion transport, as described on page 58 (see Fig. 52).

Microelectrode techniques have now been developed to such a degree of precision that differences in degree of depolarisation between one part of a neurone and another can be detected. From study of intracellular recordings Frank and Fuortes have proposed that the action spike of the motor neurone is initiated in a limited region only of the cell membrane (the region with the lowest threshold for excitation), probably at the axon hillock, from which it may be conducted to the axon without necessarily propagating a spike into the soma itself.

When the action spike is propagated to the cell body, the rising limb of the spike is seen to carry a notch about a third of the way to the summit. This notch is believed by Frank and Fuortes to represent the depolarisation of the lowest threshold section of the cell's membrane followed later by depolarisation of the soma membrane with its higher threshold for discharge.

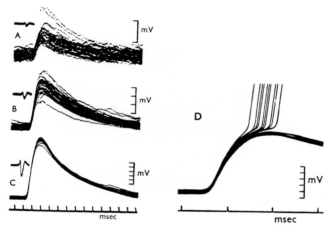

FIG. 52. POSTSYNAPTIC POTENTIALS RECORDED BY A
MICROELECTRODE FROM INSIDE A MOTOR NEURONE IN THE SPINAL
CORD OF A CAT

The responses shown were evoked monosynaptically by stimulation of the dorsal root and were recorded from an anterior horn cell. In *A*, *B* and *C* the afferent volleys were of three different strengths as indicated by their size in the insets (all recorded at the same amplification). The motor neurone responses were correspondingly graded as shown by the scales of amplification to the right of each record. All records depict the superposition of about 40 traces (positivity up). In *A*, *B* and *C* the degree of depolarisation was insufficient to trigger a spike potential. In *D* from another neurone, spikes have been generated following 10 of the stimuli and rise out of the picture.

(From Coombs, Eccles and Fatt (1955) *J. Physiol.* (*Lond.*), **130**, 374.)

Similarly, in neuro-neural synapses, axosomatic or axodendritic, the critical level of polarisation change initiated by electrotonic spread of the graded postsynaptic potential must be reached at a part of the membrane that is electrically excitable to the inward flow of current. The view held at one time that all dendrites were inexcitable, has recently had to be modified following the demonstration by Purpura, one of its former proponents, that in certain cases the dendritic systems can and do generate spikes; at the time of writing, examples so far identified include dendritic systems of hippocampal neurones; of pyramids in immature neocortex; of ventrobasal thalamic neurones; and of neurones of the brain stem reticular core.

The squid, which provided an axon large enough for the first successful insertion of an electrode for recording from the inside

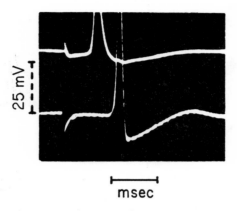

FIG. 53

Simultaneous intracellular recordings from a presynaptic fibre (upper channel) and a postsynaptic fibre (lower channel) of a squid stellate ganglion. Note synaptic delay.

(From Hagiwara and Tasaki (1958) *J. Physiol.* (*Lond.*), **143**, 114.)

of the membrane (see Fig. 26) also provided the giant synapse from which simultaneous pre- and postsynaptic potentials were first recorded by Bullock and Hagiwara. In Fig. 53 the simultaneous recording is reproduced of the presynaptic spike potential generated by chemical transmission across the synapse.

Since the postsynaptic potential increases in amplitude by summation as a result of presynaptic bombardment, the threshold for evocation of a spike is reached earlier the stronger the bombardment although the spike that is generated remains all-or-nothing in size. This is a mechanism underlying the well-known observation that latency of response increases with decrease in intensity of stimulus. An example of this recorded intracellularly was shown in Fig. 46 on page 97.

As can be seen from the illustrations, the graded postsynaptic potentials, whether excitatory or inhibitory, take some considerable time to decay. The delay is in part determined by the electrical time constant of the postsynaptic membrane (which is especially long in cold-blooded animals) and in part to residual action of transmitter at the postsynaptic membrane. This is thought to account, at least in part, for repetitive discharges in postsynaptic neurones evoked by single volleys to the presynaptic fibre.

It has been suggested by Eccles that the inhibitory transmitters may exert their effect on different regions of the soma membrane of the same recipient neurone as the excitors. His group has some evidence from their intracellular studies that the inhibitory transmitter effects the hyperpolarising of the postsynaptic membrane by transitorily increasing its permeability to chloride ions so that they rush into the cell and, being anions, raise the (negative) potential difference between the inside and the outside. At the same time there is also an increase in permeability to potassium which moves out of the cell. The departure of potassium, because it is a cation, also tends to increase the negativity of the inside of the cell. This rise in potential difference is not large, being of the order of 10 mV. A permeability change that is in effect the increase in size of the pores of a sieve would suffice, for both the K and the Cl ions are so much smaller than Na and other physiologically occurring ions.

The chemical nature of any possible inhibitory transmitters is not yet known. Since, apparently, they actively hyperpolarise the postsynaptic cell they are to be differentiated from pharmacological agents that merely block the depolarising action of excitatory transmitters. According to Grundfest, one of the blocking agents of the latter type is gamma aminobutyric acid, a product of glutamic acid metabolism. Florey and his group have identified as an active principle Factor I, an inhibitory substance that can be extracted from mammalian brain.

The transmitter at the skeletal neuromuscular junction (and other so-called cholinergic junctions) has been proved to be acetylcholine, while at adrenergic junctions it is noradrenaline. No direct identification has, however, yet been made of the transmitters at neuro-neural synapses in the mammalian brain.

TRANSMISSION ACROSS THE NEUROMUSCULAR
JUNCTION

Electron microscopy has revealed the structure of a neuro-muscular junction to consist of a deeply-folded postsynaptic muscle end-plate, surrounding (in section) the almost circular presynaptic nerve fibre terminals. The nerve membrane is not

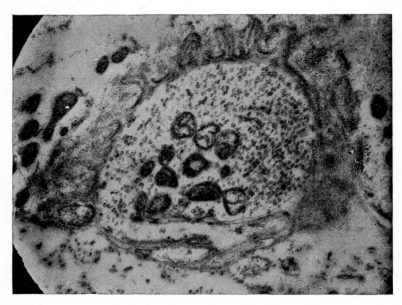

FIG. 54. ULTRASTRUCTURE OF A NEUROMUSCULAR JUNCTION
(LIZARD) AS REVEALED BY THE ELECTRON MICROSCOPE

A single terminal axon is seen in cross-section lying invaginated in the muscle fibre and surrounded by junctional folds of the muscle membrane. Mitochondria appear in both the axoplasm of the nerve and the sarcoplasm of the muscle as dark bodies of round or oval shape. Within the axoplasm the other smaller bodies, less dense in their centres, are the vesicles referred to in the text. Magnification: × 70,000.

(This photograph has been provided through the kindness of Dr J. David Robertson.)

in contact with the surfaces of the folds but with the base from which they rise, and is nowhere more than 1 μ distant from the postsynaptic membrane. The structure of a junction can be seen in Fig. 54 which reproduces one of Robertson's electron micrographs.

Since 1936, when Dale and his colleagues first discovered that acetylcholine is released from the endings of the terminal fibres of active motor nerves, much new knowledge has been added by subsequent workers. Nachmansohn discovered that a specific enzyme (cholinesterase) was present in high concentrations at the junction, limiting the effect of acetylcholine by hydrolysis and thus controlling it. Any inhibitor of this specific cholinesterase (such as eserine) preserves the acetylcholine and prolongs its action, whereas its effect is prevented by any blocking agent that acts on the postsynaptic membrane (e.g. curare).

The electrical theory that transmission across the neuromuscular junction is effected by current flow from the nerve terminals has lost ground since the work of Kuffler with microelectrodes. He devised a technique that demonstrated quite clearly that subliminal currents that set up electrotonic potentials in the nerve do not cross to the muscle end-plate. Moreover, supraliminal currents that evoke a spike potential in the nerve do not set up synchronous potentials in the end-plate (as one would expect from an electrical field effect), but take at least a millisecond to evoke transmission. During this millisecond, acetylcholine is released from the nerve endings and diffuses across the gap, one micron wide, to act on the postsynaptic membrane. Even in the 'resting' condition, i.e. when no propagated impulse is passing down the nerve, minute amounts of acetylcholine are released at its terminals, not continously, but in 'quanta' containing many molecules. These quanta have been shown by Fatt and Katz to evoke tiny non-propagated postsynaptic potentials in the muscle end-plate. The mechanism of release of acetylcholine at the nerve endings has not yet been fully elucidated, but it is known to be blocked by excess magnesium and by calcium lack. There is evidence that the vesicular structures seen by electron microscopy (Fig. 54) contain quanta of acetylcholine and are hence closely related to this secretory process.

The electrical potential set up in the postsynaptic membrane by acetylcholine that has diffused across the gap is known as the *end-plate potential*. This is a local depolarisation that, according to the findings of Nastuk, is apparently produced, not by penetration into the postsynaptic membrane by acetylcholine ions themselves, but by a general increase in permeability. The current flow derives from the postsynaptic element and is not a spread of current from the nerve. With subliminal excitation (too weak to evoke an action potential in the muscle fibre) this increase in permeability lasts only a few milliseconds; its electrical sign is an increase of internal negativity, rising during the active diffusion of acetylcholine and falling off when the acetylcholine is hydrolysed by the waiting cholinesterase. The decay of the end-plate potential follows an exponential time course and its time-constant furnishes some information about the resistance-capacitance network of the membrane through which it leaks away. Spatially, the end-plate potential decays also approximately exponentially from the point of stimulation and cannot be detected at a distance of more than a few millimetres along the fibre.

The end-plate potential is an example of a graded response; it has no refractory period, and subsequent excitation before it has decayed will cause summation along the whole length of its electrotonic extension (i.e. a few mm). When the summed end-plate potentials reach a certain threshold (approximately 30 mV) an action spike develops that is propagated along the muscle fibre. Figure 55 from Kuffler illustrates a propagated action spike rising from a non-propagated end-plate potential and the blocking action on it of curare. Just as in a nerve (see page 58), the rising phase of the spike is accompanied by a brief increase in permeability, specifically to sodium which rushes in, swinging the internal potential from negativity through zero to positivity (an overshoot of approximately 50 μV). The membrane is thus rendered refractory to a second impulse during the time that it takes for restoration of sufficient internal negativity to trip off a second spike. As in the nerve action potential, that of the muscle fibre also has a period of increased permeability to potassium that follows the rise of the spike. There is evidence that the sodium-specific permeability changes that give rise to the spike originate in areas of the post-synaptic membrane adjacent to, but not identical with, the point of origin of the end-plate potential, i.e. along its electro-tonic extension in the muscle fibre.

Neuromuscular transmission differs from synaptic trans-mission between nerve cells in anatomical structure. The nerve ending, bare of myelin, branches over the end-plate of the

muscle fibre; at this junction the impulse in the nerve is transmitted, after a delay, to the muscle fibres (Fig. 56).

By means of focal recordings with microelectrodes at the
terminal branches of motor neurones at the end-plate of
the muscle fibre, Katz and Miledi have been able to obtain

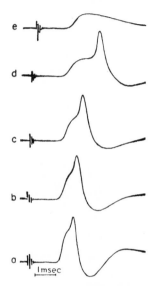

FIG. 55. POTENTIAL EVOKED AT THE END-PLATE OF A SINGLE
MUSCLE FIBRE BY STIMULATION OF THE NERVE

Stimulation occurred at the break in the line.
In the lowest record (a) the end-plate potential can be seen with the
consequent muscle spike rising from it. In (b), (c), (d) and (e), curare was
added and progressively blocked the muscle response. In (e) the end-plate
potential alone remains, all neuromuscular transmission having been
blocked by the curare.

(From Kuffler (1942) *J. Neurophysiol.*, **5**, 18.)

direct measures of the delay at the neuromuscular junction in
the frog and have demonstrated the direct facilitating action of
calcium ions on the release of acetylcholine by the nerve
impulse.

In summary then, just as in excited nerve where the non-
propagated postsynaptic potential precedes the conducted
action spike, so at the neuromuscular junction a non-propagated
end-plate potential precedes the action potential of the muscle

fibre. The local postsynaptic potential in nerve and the end-plate potential at the neuromuscular junction have electrotonic effects, decaying exponentially in space and time. Neither is

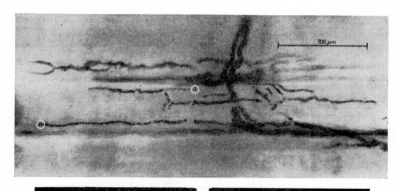

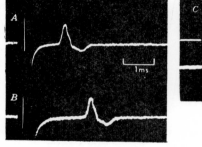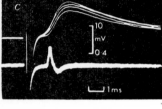

FIG. 56. MOTOR NEURONE TERMINALS

Above: Micrograph of the frog motor neurone terminal, stimulation of which at points *A* and *B* evoked the responses reproduced on the left, below.
Below: On left, antidromic nerve spike evoked by extracellular focal stimulation at *A* (upper trace) of a non-myelinated terminal 14 μ from the myelinated parent fibre, and at *B* (lower trace) 230 μ distant.
On right, from another fibre, the antidromic nerve spike evoked by stimulation of a nerve terminal and the intracellularly recorded end-plate potential.
(From Katz and Miledi (1965) *Proc. roy. Soc. B.*, **161,** 453.)

propagated, and each represents a local depolarisation. Each is capable of summation, provided a second impulse is received before total decay of the electrotonus set up by the first. In each case if the electrotonic potentials reach a critical threshold at excitable membrane a propagated impulse is evoked.

Since the action potential of the muscle fibre follows the

all-or-nothing law, intensity of response depends, as Sherrington concluded, on the number of activated synapses.

BIBLIOGRAPHY

Brock, L. C., Coombs, J. S. and Eccles, J. R. (1952) The recording of potentials from motoneurones with an intracellular electrode. *J. Physiol. (Lond.)*, **117**, 431–460.

Bronk, D. (1939) Synaptic mechanisms in sympathetic ganglia. *J. Neurophysiol.*, **2**, 380–401.

Bullock, T. H. and Hagiwara, S. (1957) Intracellular recording from the giant synapse of the squid. *J. gen. Physiol.*, **40**, 565–577.

Coombs, J. S., Eccles, J. D. and Fatt, P. (1955) The specific ionic conductances and the ionic movements across the motoneural membrane that produce the inhibitory post-synaptic potential. *J. Physiol. (Lond.)*, **130**, 326–373.

Coombs, J. S., Eccles, J. C. and Fatt, P. (1955) Excitatory synaptic action in motoneurones. *J. Physiol. (Lond.)*, **130**, 374–395.

Dale, H. H., Feldberg, W. and Vogt, M. (1936) Release of acetylcholine at voluntary motor nerve endings. *J. Physiol. (Lond.)*, **86**, 353–380.

Del Castillo, J. and Katz, B. (1956) Biophysical aspects of neuromuscular transmission. *Progr. Biophys.*, **6**, 121–170.

Eccles, J. C. (1957) *The Physiology of Nerve Cells*. Johns Hopkins Press.

Eccles, J. C., Fatt, P. and Koketsu, K. (1953) Cholinergic and inhibitory synapses in a central nervous pathway. *Australian J. Sci.*, **16**, 50–54.

Eccles, J. C. (1946) Synaptic potentials of motoneurones. *J. Neurophysiol.*, **9**, 87–120.

Eccles, J. C. (1964) *The Physiology of Synapses*. Springer-Verlag, Berlin.

Eccles, R. M. (1955) Intracellular potentials recorded from a mammalian sympathetic ganglia. *J. Physiol. (Lond.)*, **130**, 572–584.

Fatt, P. and Katz, B. (1952) Spontaneous subthreshold activity at motor nerve endings. *J. Physiol. (Lond.)*, **117**, 109–128.

Fatt, P. and Katz, B. (1951) An analysis of the end-plate potential recorded with an intracellular electrode. *J. Physiol. (Lond.)*, **115**, 320–370.

Forbes, A. (1922) The interpretation of spinal reflexes in terms of present knowledge of nerve conduction. *Physiol. Rev.*, **2**, 361–414.

Freygang, W. H. and Frank, K. (1959) Extracellular potentials from single spinal motoneurones. *J. gen. Physiol.*, **42**, 749–760.

Fuortes, M. G. F., Frank, K. and Becker, M. C. (1957) Steps in the production of motoneuron spikes. *J. gen. Physiol.*, **40**, 735–752.

Grundfest, H. (1957) Electrical inexcitability of synapses and some consequences in the central nervous system. *Physiol. Rev.*, **37**, 337–361.

Hagiwara, S. and Tasaki, I. (1958) A study of the mechanism of impulse transmission across the giant synapse of the squid. *J. Physiol. (Lond.)*, **143**, 114–137.

Katz, B. (1962) The transmission of impulses from nerve to muscle, and the subcellular unit of synaptic action. *Proc. roy. Soc. B.*, **155**, 455–479.

Katz, B. and Miledi, R. (1965) Propagation of electric activity in motor nerve terminals. *Proc. roy. Soc. B.*, **161**, 453–482.

Katz, B. and Miledi, R. (1965) The measurement of synaptic delay, and the time course of acetylcholine release at the neuromuscular junction. *Proc. roy. Soc. B.*, **161**, 483–495.

Katz, B. and Miledi, R. (1965) The effect of calcium on acetylcholine release from motor nerve terminals. *Proc. roy. Soc. B.*, **161**, 496–503.

Kuffler, S. W. (1942) Electric potential changes at an isolated nerve-muscle junction. *J. Neurophysiol.*, **5**, 18–26.

Kuffler, S. W. (1942) Responses during refractory period at myoneural junction in isolated nerve-muscle fibre preparation. *J. Neurophysiol.*, **5**, 199–209.

Kuffler, S. W. (1949) Transmitter mechanism at the nerve-muscle junction. *Arch. Sci. physiol.*, **3**, 585–601.

Libet, B. (1965) 'Slow synaptic responses in autonomic ganglia.' In *Studies in Physiology*. Springer-Verlag, New York.

Lorente de Nó, R. (1939) Transmission of impulses through cranial motor nuclei. *J. Neurophysiol.*, **2**, 402–472.

McLennan, H. (1963) *Synaptic Transmission*. Saunders, Philadelphia.

Nastuk, W. M. (1953) The electrical activity of the muscle cell membrane at the neuromuscular junction. *J. cell. comp. Physiol.*, **42**, 249–272.

Robertson, J. D. (1956) The ultrastructure of a reptilian myoneural junction. *J. biophys. biochem. Cytol.*, **2**, 381–394.

Sanders, F. K. and Young, J. Z. (1940) Learning and other functions of the higher nervous centres of sepia. *J. Neurophysiol.*, **3**, 501–526.

Sherrington, C. S. (1947) *Integrative Action of the Nervous System*, 2nd ed. Cambridge University Press.

Tauc, L. (1962) Site of origin and propagation of spike in the giant neuron of *Aplysia*. *J. gen. Physiol.*, **45**, 1099–1115.

The Electrical Potentials of the Spinal Cord

THE classic studies on the spinal cord by the pioneers of the 1930s and 1940s were all carried out with gross electrodes placed either on the surface of the cord or on the dorsal and ventral roots. From this work evolved our basic knowledge of the monosynaptic reflex, of polysynaptic connexions and of the long pathways in the cord.

With the advent of the newer knowledge gained by the use of intracellular electrodes and the increasing understanding of excitatory and inhibitory postsynaptic potentials, as described in the previous chapter, some of the earlier findings can now be understood at the cellular level, including the slow potentials that long outlast the presynaptic stimulus.

With gross electrodes it was observed many years ago that a shower of discharges could be recorded from a ventral root following a single brief stimulus to the dorsal root of the same segment.

Forbes framed the original proposition that this after-discharge might be the effect of long delay paths; this hypothesis suggests that, in spinal reflexes, the signals initiated in the sensory nerve reach the motor nerves by multiple paths with differing numbers of interneurones having varied conduction rates, each also contributing some synaptic delay, so that a long shower of stimuli to the final motor neurone results from a single afferent shock (see Fig. 57).

Interneurones lie entirely within the central nervous system. Those of the cord are found in the grey matter from just below the dorsal surface to the lower edge of the ventral horn. All do not serve the same function, some being excitatory and some apparently inhibitory. Until the development of techniques for recording from inside the spinal cord by means of micro-electrodes, the electrical properties of neurones lying wholly

within the cord had to be inferred from external recordings—
from Gasser's intermediary potentials (page 120), from the
dorsal root potentials (page 122), and from studies of polysynaptic reflexes (see below).

Starting with Renshaw in 1940, many workers have explored
these small internuncial neurones more directly with microelectrodes (outside the cells) and some knowledge of them is

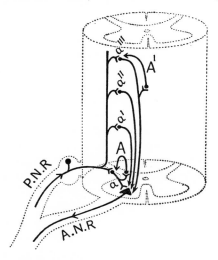

FIG. 57. DIAGRAMMATIC REPRESENTATION OF DELAY PATHS AND
SELF RE-EXCITING CIRCUITS IN THE SPINAL CORD

Pathways are shown for a sensory impulse entering by the dorsal root
(P.N.R.) and travelling through any of four interneurones (a, a', a'' and a''')
at different segmental levels. In this diagram the delay would be due
only to the longer conducting path. Forbes's hypothesis postulates a
greater number of interneurones, and hence of synaptic delays, in the
longer paths. Two re-exciting circuits, A and A', are also shown. The
common final motor neurone lies in the ventral horn and its axon leaves
the cord by the ventral root (A.N.R.).

(From Samson Wright (1965) *Applied Biology*. Oxford University Press.)

beginning to accumulate. Many workers have now succeeded
in penetrating interneurones with a fine electrode and have
recorded from the inside of their cell bodies. One of their outstanding properties is that they have higher discharge frequencies than the anterior horn cells whose function is to innervate
slowly-moving muscles; they also respond to incoming stimuli
too weak to fire the motor neurones. Their influence in the

neuronal pool can therefore be a subtly graded one, for most of these rapidly discharging cells receive impulses from many afferent sources and connect synaptically with many efferent neurones on which they can exert influence through subliminal changes.

Ventral Root Potentials. When recording electrodes are placed on a ventral root, the response to stimulation of the dorsal root at the same segment is a spike which appears after one synaptic delay—that of the synapse between the dorsal root fibre and the ventral horn cell. Following this is a shower of irregular potentials. Figure 58 shows such discharges recorded by Eccles from a ventral root of a cat when the dorsal root of the same segment was stimulated by a single volley. The spike is the composite response of the motor components of the two-neurone arc, *the monosynaptic reflex*, and the subsequent potentials are the responses of the same motor neurones to stimuli arriving later via the internuncial neurones; in the record they are separated from the spike by the time consumed at the intermediate synapses. They are themselves spike potentials in origin but have become dispersed in time.

The figure shows, additionally, the effect of barbiturate on these ventral root potentials which gradually die out until finally only the synaptic potential remains.

The physiological counterpart of this artificially-stimulated synaptic reflex is the myotatic or stretch reflex, as exemplified by the knee jerk. The sensory end-organ is the annulo-spiral muscle spindle and the afferent inflow is predominantly in the largest fibres of lowest threshold, the Group Ia* afferents with diameters above 12 μ that have a conduction velocity of 60 to 120 m/sec. Muscle spindles have also some more slowly conducting afferents with rates between 30 and 50 m/sec.

Lloyd further analysed these reflex pathways by studying the activity in the ventral root following stimulation not only at the dorsal root but also of the sensory nerves from the muscles and skin. He found that the afferents from the skin are fibres of higher threshold than those from the muscle spindles and carry the impulses primarily responsible for the discharges

---

* In this terminology, the numeral indicates the size range (and hence the conduction velocity) of the fibre, and the letter its function. Group Ia afferents come from muscle spindles, Group Ib from Golgi tendon organs. They differ in function but not in size.

through the delay paths (Fig. 59). The spike discharge of the
two-neurone arc is predominantly, though not entirely, restricted to the motor neurones of the same muscle whose spindles

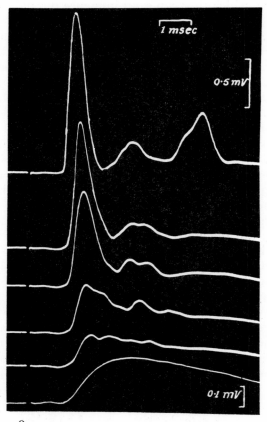

FIG. 58. DISCHARGES IN A VENTRAL ROOT FOLLOWING
STIMULATION OF THE DORSAL ROOT OF THE SAME SEGMENT (CAT)

The initial spike response of the two-neurone is arc followed by the irregular
discharges arriving via the polyneuronal pathways. Top curve unanaesthetised; lower curves show effect of increasing depth of barbiturate
anaesthesia until only the synaptic potential remains (bottom curve).

(From Eccles (1946) *J. Neurophysiol.*, **9**, 87.)

have been stretched, whereas discharges through the polyneuronal arc appear also in neighbouring motor nerves to
closely-associated muscles. For example, stimulation of the

tibial nerve (of the posterior tibial muscle) produces delayed
reflex discharges in the peroneal nerve to the anterior tibial

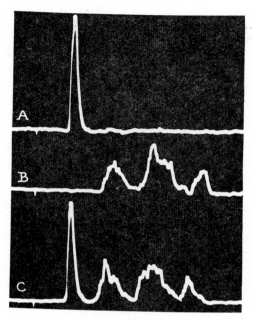

FIG. 59. DISCHARGES IN A VENTRAL ROOT FOLLOWING STIMULATION
OF DIFFERENT AFFERENT NERVES

A : Initial spike response of the two-neurone arc evoked by stimulation
of nerve from a muscle.
B : Delayed discharges arriving via polyneuronal pathways from stimulation of a sensory nerve from the skin.
C : Stimulation of a dorsal root resulting in activation both of the monosynaptic and the polysynaptic routes.
(From Lloyd (1943) *J. Neurophysiol.*, **6**, 293.)

muscle, but no trace of the direct monosynaptic discharge is
found anywhere but in the posterior tibial muscle itself.

Lloyd has shown that afferents from a given muscle mediate
excitation in the motor neurones of that same muscle (via the
two-neurone arc), facilitate action in its synergists at the same
joint, and inhibit its antagonists at that joint. For example, in
the thigh, excitation of the nerve from the quadriceps inhibits
the biceps semitendinosus and vice versa. There is a difference
of opinion as to whether the inhibitory pathway is monosynaptic

or whether it includes an interneurone with special inhibitory properties. More recent views of inhibition in the spinal cord are given in a later section (see page 125).

The monosynaptic response of the motor neurone when recorded from inside the cell shows the initial graded excitatory postsynaptic potential described in the previous chapter, and Eccles has shown that this can be recorded also from the ventral root of the segment whose dorsal root is being stimulated. This is known as *ventral root electrotonus.*

Cord Dorsum Potentials. Before investigators had succeeded in recording from within anterior horn cells and interneurones, many of the characteristics of transmission within the cord were inferred from the potentials recordable from its surface and from its roots.

In 1933 Gasser and Graham demonstrated that, when an afferent spinal root is stimulated by a single shock, the response recordable from the surface of the cord is a spike followed some time later by slower irregular potentials. The response is recordable beyond the segment stimulated. The spike in this case is the action potential of the long axons of the dorsal root neurones which run up in the dorsal columns of the spinal cord. It follows the stimulus with very little delay—in fact only the delay due to the conduction time of the fibres involved. The spike potential is characteristically triphasic in form, as are all axon potentials recorded *in situ* by longitudinally orientated electrodes, and has the same temporal characteristics as the action spike of mammalian A fibres, with a spike duration of 0·5 msec.

With the recording electrodes placed directly on the surface of the spinal cord in this way, rather than on the roots, Gasser found that the action spike of the intraspinal sensory fibres was followed by a slow negative potential and then by a long-lasting positive component (positive in that the recording electrode nearer to the stimulated root was positive to the more distant one). These potentials were named by Gasser *the intermediary cord potentials* (see Fig. 60).

Various interpretations have been given of the slow positive component that follows the spike: that it represented the discharge of internuncial neurones (Gasser); that it represented persisting depolarisation in the terminal branches of the dorsal

root fibres (Barron and Matthews); and that it was caused by
a complex consisting of activity in afferent terminals followed

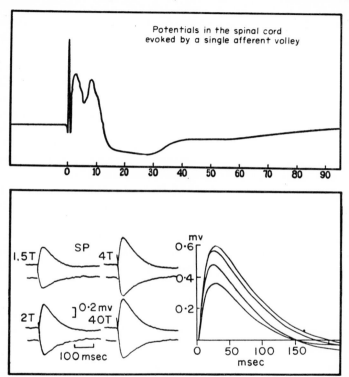

FIG. 60. POTENTIALS OF THE SPINAL CORD EVOKED BY STIMULATION
OF A DORSAL ROOT

Above: Gasser's classic recording with gross electrodes on the dorsal surface
of the cord.
(From Gasser (1937) *Harvey Lect.*, **32**, 169.)

Below: Microelectrode recordings from inside the fibre at four different
strengths of stimulation (T = threshold for response). Upper trace shows
a long-lasting negative dorsal root potential and the lower trace the
similarly long-lasting positive cord dorsum potential.

(From Eccles, Kostyuk and Schmidt (1962) *J. Physiol.* (*Lond.*), **161,** 237.)

by the discharge of cell bodies of interneurones (McCouch and
Austin).

The more recent development of microelectrodes able to
penetrate neurones has, however, shown these slow potentials

to be in large part postsynaptic potentials generated in the groups of motorneurones and interneurones invaded by the dorsal root fibres, only a fraction being accounted for by persisting activity in dorsal root terminals. In fact, the mechanism is apparently identical with that involved in the slow components of dorsal root potentials.

Dorsal Root Potentials. Another type of long-lasting potential change was revealed by the discovery by the Umraths and by Barron and Matthews (since confirmed by Eccles, Bremer and others) of long-persisting potential changes having the properties of electrotonic potentials (see page 79). In recording externally from dorsal roots rather than from the spinal cord itself, these workers found the spike response to stimulation of the same sensory root to be followed by slow negative potential changes lasting about 0·2 sec in the cat and longer still in the frog (see Fig. 61). These potentials were found to exhibit temporal and spatial summation and, in contrast to spike potentials, to show a decrement with distance similar to the decay of electrotonus (see page 80). If the stimulating electrodes are placed on the central end of a cut dorsal root, the slow potentials can be recorded from the adjacent dorsal roots without the immediately-conducted spike of the root fibres. They were interpreted by Barron and Matthews as being due to depolarisation of the fine terminal fibres of collaterals from the dorsal column axons, but they are now known to be postsynaptic in origin as first suggested by Bonnet and Bremer. These slow potentials owe their time-course to the characteristics of synapses and not of axons or cell discharges.

A detailed analysis of the sequence of dorsal root potential changes was made by Lloyd and McIntyre who showed that the slow potential of Barron and Matthews is, in the unstimulated neighbouring roots, preceded by four other potential swings. These are illustrated in Fig. 62. Of these, the first, second and third (DR. I negative, DR. II positive, DR. III negative at the electrode nearer to the spinal cord) were interpreted as the electrotonic spread, from the cord back into the root, of the triphasic spike potential of the dorsal column fibres (which has already been described on page 120 and illustrated in Fig. 60).

This type of electrotonus set up in neighbouring fibres by

the external currents of action potentials in active fibres has been described in Chapter 6 and is illustrated in Figs. 31 and

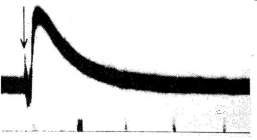

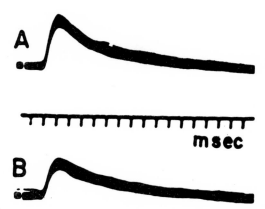

FIG. 61. POTENTIAL CHANGES IN AN INTACT DORSAL ROOTLET

Above: Barron and Matthews's classic picture of the response to a single shock to the afferent nerve as recorded with gross external electrodes. Time signal: 10 msec.

(From Barron and Matthews (1938) *J. Physiol. (Lond.)*, **92**, 276.)

Below: Intracellularly recorded excitatory postsynaptic potential generated monosynaptically by stimulation of the afferent nerve.

(From Eccles (1957) *The Physiology of Nerve Cells.* Johns Hopkins Press.)

32. It will be noted that the sign of the electrotonic potential is of opposite polarity to the action potential which caused it, as will immediately be clear from a study of the sinks and sources of current in Fig. 31. In the stimulated root these first

three spikes are replaced by the diphasic (positive-negative) spike typical of active fibres.

The fourth component, DR. IV, a slower potential, negative in the stimulated root, positive in its neighbours, was originally thought by Lloyd to be caused by residual activity in the terminal fibres both of the presynaptic axons which form the intraspinal collaterals from the dorsal root and (but to a lesser degree) of interneurones within the core. This view is not shared by Eccles who, from his intracellular records from the cell bodies of motor neurones, holds this long-lasting potential to

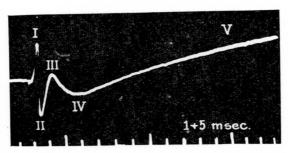

FIG. 62. SEQUENCE OF POTENTIAL CHANGES RECORDED FROM A DORSAL ROOT ADJACENT TO THE ROOT STIMULATED (BULL-FROG)
For explanation see text.
(From Lloyd and McIntyre (1949) *J. gen. Physiol.*, **32**, 409.)

be wholly postsynaptic in origin. He regards the currents generated in the postsynaptic neurones as depolarising, in turn, the dorsal root fibres which come into contract with them. This phenomenon of the slow graded potential in the dorsal roots is what is known as *dorsal root electrotonus*.

Some of the interpretations made by inference from external recordings of the kind just described will no doubt undergo modification as more information accumulates from the newer techniques by which recordings are being made from electrodes penetrating, not only the cell bodies and the axons of the motor neurones of the spinal cord, but also the much smaller inter-neurones and the dorsal root fibres. An example is the report by Frank and Fuortes that they could find no counterpart of the slow electrotonic potentials of dorsal or ventral roots when they recorded from the interior of the root fibres themselves.

Their intra-axonal recording did, however, confirm the existence, at least in the laboratory setting, of dorsal root reflexes.

Dorsal Root Reflexes. In addition to the apparent electrotonic spread out along dorsal roots after they have been stimulated there are also conducted impulses passing out in an antidromic direction. These are the *dorsal root reflexes* first observed by Horsley and Gotch in 1891 and later re-discovered in 1934 by Matthews, and studied by Barron and Matthews, and by Toennies. They are usually seen as spikes riding on the contour of the D.R.V. wave. That they are indeed antidromic impulses in the afferent dorsal root fibres (and not the activity of efferent fibres) has been shown by Frank and Fuortes's finding that both the evoking impulse and the reflex response can on occasion be detected consecutively in the same fibre by use of an inserted microelectrode. The outgoing impulses follow the ingoing ones that evoke them by an interval that is never less that 2·5 msec and may be as long as 15 msec. If dorsal root reflexes occur naturally (as well as in the experimental situation) it would seem that their function is probably a control over input. As Frank has pointed out, over-stimulation of a receptor would result in some impulses never reaching the cord since they would find some fibres already occupied by the outgoing reflex discharge.

Inhibition in the Spinal Cord. Direct inhibition (which should be distinguished from the failure of excitatory impulses to fire a neurone during its refractory period) has been the subject of considerable study by Eccles and his group using fine intracellular electrodes (see Fig. 49). From these studies Eccles views inhibition as being mediated by short-axoned interneurones within the ventral horn of the spinal cord, although attempts to support this view by anatomical evidence have been unsuccessful. No short-axoned cells could be found by the Scheibels in the ventral horns of either rodents or cats. It seems likely that the anatomical substrate of the electrophysiological findings lies in other elements.

According to the hypothesis of Eccles, those interneurones which function as inhibitors of motor neurones secrete a different chemical transmitter from those which function as excitors. The difference in action of the transmitters is that the inhibitory ones cause a hyperpolarisation of the ventral horn cell, whereas the excitatory transmitters cause a depolarisation. There is no evidence that any one neurone can secrete both types of transmitter. According to this hypothesis, it is the identity of the interneurones in the path that decides whether the outcome is to be excitation or inhibition in the final common path. In the past a clear distinction has sometimes not been made between this type of inhibition and the subnormality conditioned by preceding activity of a cell. These are two different phenomena. Lloyd has called the first of these *direct inhibition* and the second, *indirect inhibition*.

In the spinal cord several types of direct inhibition have been differentiated by Eccles, all acting through hyperpolarisation of the motor neurones. The principal ones as defined by him are: disynaptic inhibition of motor neurones by large (Group I*a*) afferents from annulo-spiral endings in antagonistic muscles (see Fig. 63); disynaptic inhibition of synergists by Group I*b* afferents from Golgi tendon organs (through interneurones in the dorsal horn); and disynaptic inhibition via the Renshaw interneurones in the ventral horn stimulated by recurrent collaterals from the motor neurones. In addition one must recognise polysynaptic inhibition of flexor reflexes through more than one interneurone set up by impulses in skin afferents, and polysynaptic inhibition by the fine Group III muscle afferents.

The first type (inhibition through Group I*a* afferents), is held by Lloyd to be monosynaptic, for he finds insufficient time for an interneurone. McCouch and Eccles, on the other hand, conclude each from his own experiments that an interneurone lies on the path. This interneurone has been located in the intermediate nucleus in the grey matter at approximately the level of the central canal, and is activated by an intermedullary collateral of the dorsal root afferent. Although this conclusion was reached from observation of time-relations and spatial mapping of potential fields, it tallies with the hypothesis that for inhibition there must be, playing on to the ventral horn cell, the type of interneurone whose terminals secrete an inhibitory transmitter. Were the pathway to be monosynaptic this would entail the terminals of the dorsal root fibres secreting both excitatory and inhibitory transmitters, though this is not entirely impossible.

In the stretch reflex reciprocal innervation has a double character. Afferents from the muscle spindles signal when the muscle is being stretched and act to inhibit contraction in the antagonist muscles and to facilitate it in their own, whereas afferents from Golgi tendon organs signal contraction and act to inhibit their attached muscles and excite the antagonists. The latter is in the second category of direct inhibition listed above. Mention has been made above of Renshaw cells as representing a third type of direct inhibition. These interneurones were named for their discoverer who died of poliomyelitis in 1946.

Renshaw cells may reach a discharge frequency as high as 1,500/sec, and they are thought by Eccles to serve a purely inhibitory action via short axons. The existence of such short-axoned cells in the ventral horn, however, still lacks anatomical evidence. The studies of Scheibel have revealed that all the cells in the ventro-medial aspect of the horn appear to be commissural cells whose long axons cross to the other side of the cord. On the other hand, the existence of recurrent collaterals from the axons of motor neurones has been known to anatomists since Golgi's demonstration of them in 1886, and Cajal's later studies of them.

In the case of the excitatory transmitter secreted by the terminals of the axon collateral there is some evidence that this may be acetylcholine. This would not really be surprising since the main axon terminals of the same neurones are known to secrete acetylcholine at the neuromuscular junction which they innervate. It seems probable that there may be several excitatory transmitters in the central nervous system, of which acetylcholine is only one. The nature of the inhibitory transmitter is unknown.

An early observation in studies of the monosynaptic reflex was that rapid repetitive stimulation of the afferent nerve evoked a larger than usual action potential postsynaptically in the motor neurone; this is known as post-tetanic potentiation and is a phenomenon invoked by some as the basis for a hypothesis that repeated use causes a permanent facilitation of synaptic transmission, a concept that has on occasion even been extended to explain memory and learning. The experimental evidence, however, indicates that post-tetanic potentiation is, as Lloyd

originally affirmed, a transient and not a permanent phenomenon. With the more direct methods of intracellular recording, the increase in spike height has been shown to be a transient

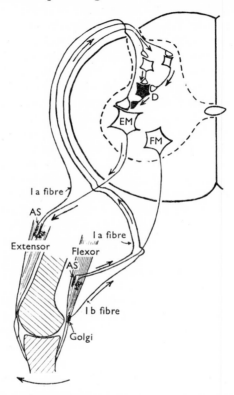

FIG. 63. ECCLES'S SCHEMATIC DIAGRAM OF SUGGESTED PATHWAYS
FOR PRESYNAPTIC INHIBITION

The small black interneurone is depicted as forming a synapse on to the
terminal of a dorsal root fibre, thereby inhibiting the excitatory action of
this presynaptic contact with the motor neurone.
AS = annulo-spiral ending. EM and FM represent extensor and flexor
motor neurones.

(From Eccles, Kostyuk and Schmidt (1962) *J. Physiol. (Lond.)*, **161,** 237.)

after-hyperpolarisation of the afferent nerve terminals that can
be mimicked by artificially hyperpolarising the nerve endings
with an applied current.

Presynaptic Inhibition. Microelectrode recordings by Frank

and Fuortes from single motor neurones revealed a type of inhibition in the spinal cord that had not previously been defined.
They found that afferent volleys could decrease the size of the
excitatory postsynaptic potential in the motor neurone without
any development of hyperpolarisation or involvement of an
interneurone. This phenomenon has received extensive study
from Eccles and his group, who reject Frank's original hypothesis that this type of inhibition is being exerted on a remote
part of the motor neurone, i.e. the dendrite, where intracellular
evidence for hyperpolarisation would be difficult to obtain. Instead, Eccles has accumulated evidence in support of his theory
that the inhibition is presynaptic and that it develops in the
terminals of the afferent fibres before they make contact with
the motor neurone. This type of presynaptic depolarisation is
identical with that postulated for the dorsal root potentials and
cord dorsum potentials described above. In other words, it is
a depolarisation of primary afferents resulting, presumably, in a
reduction of the transmitter output from the presynaptic
terminals. Figure 63 is the schema drawn by Eccles to illustrate
his concept of presynaptic inhibition.

Innervation of Muscle and the Gamma Efferent System. Although
there are some species differences, there are, in general, two
types of sensory receptor in the muscle itself, the annulo-spiral
endings winding round the central part of the muscle spindles
formed by intrafusal fibres, and the fine flower-sprays often
found at either end of the spindle. A third type of sensory
receptor lies, not in the muscle fibre, but at the insertion of the
tendon into the muscle; this is the Golgi tendon organ (see
Fig. 64).

The annulo-spiral endings are served by the large Group IA
fibres that are responsible for the excitation of the extensors of
the monosynaptic reflex and (via interneurones) for inhibition
of the antagonists.

The flower-spray receptors are served by much finer fibres,
namely Group II and III, and serve the flexor reflexes, i.e. they
lead to excitation of the flexors and to inhibition of the extensors.

It is the Golgi endings, located in the insertion of tendons
into the muscle, that signal degree of tension in extensor muscles.
The tendons have no motor innervation. When the muscle
contracts and the spindle shortens, it ceases to fire discharges up

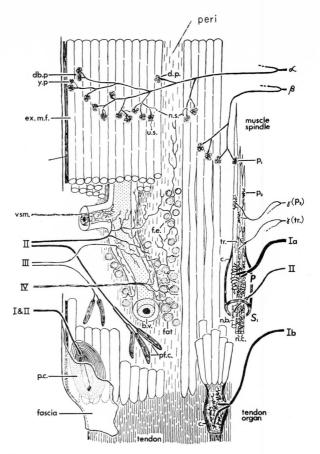

FIG. 64. SCHEMA OF THE INNERVATION OF MAMMALIAN SKELETAL
MUSCLE BASED ON A STUDY OF THE CAT

Those nerve fibres shown on the right of the diagram are exclusively
concerned with muscle innervation; those on the left also take part in the
innervation of other tissues. Roman numerals refer to the groups of
myelinated (I, II, III) and unmyelinated (IV) sensory fibres; Greek
letters refer to motor fibres. Features of terminal sprouting and degeneration are omitted from the spindle. *b.v.*, blood vessel; *c.*, capsule; *db.p.*,
double motor end-plate; *d.p.*, degenerating end-plate; *epi.*, epimysium;
ex.m.f., extrafusal muscle film; *n.b.*, nuclear-bag intrafusal muscle fibre;
n.c., nuclear-chain intrafusal muscle fibre; *n.s.*, nodal sprout; *p*, primary
ending; p_1, p_2, two types of intrafusal end-plates; *peri.*, perimysium;
p.c., Pacinian corpuscle; *pf.c.*, paciniform corpuscle; s_1, secondary
ending; *tr.*, trail ending; *u.s.*, ultraterminal sprout; *vsm*, vasomotor fibres;
v.p., young motor end-plate ('accessory ending').

(By courtesy of Dr D. Barker, Ciba Symposium, 1967.)

its sensory nerve. The contraction, however, pulls on the tendon and the Golgi organ, previously silent, then begins to fire (see Fig. 65).

Stemming from the original observations made by Leksell in Stockholm in 1945, a previously unproven reflex control of muscle stretch came to light. This is mediated by the fine

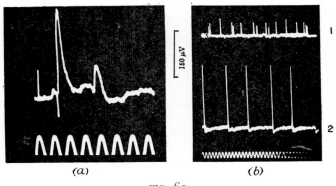

(a)   (b)

FIG. 65

(a) Response of a single large motor fibre (15 μ) followed by that of gamma efferents (5 μ) in a ventral root filament (cat). Conduction distance 11 cm. Time line: 1,000 c/s. Amplitude calibration to right of photograph. (b) Microelectrode recordings from a ventral root filament containing one large motor fibre and some gamma efferents (cat): (1) At rest, showing discharge from gamma fibres only. (2) During stretch, showing inhibition of discharge from gamma efferents and excitation in the single large fibre.
(From Hunt (1951) *J. Physiol. (Lond.)*, **115**, 456.)

efferent fibres running out from the spinal cord to the muscle spindles themselves and constituting (as measured in cats and monkey) about one-third of the ventral root outflow to the limbs.

The diameters of gamma fibres in the cat lie between 3 and 8 μ in contrast with those of the axons of the large motor neurones which are above 12 μ. As long ago as 1934, O'Leary, Heinbecker and Bishop had suggested that these small myelinated fibres might innervate muscle spindles, a suggestion now fully proved by the work of the Stockholm school, and by the detailed analyses of Hunt and Kuffler and others. The muscle spindle efferent system is under control from higher centres in the brain stem, cerebrum and cerebellum, and is one of several examples of centrifugal control of input to the nervous system exerted at the level of the receptor as is described later in this book (see pages 162, 178 and 204).

That a degree of control of this kind may operate in the central nervous system was many times suggested before its anatomical substrate was discovered. In fact, the suggestion goes back at least as far as Charles Bell who, in 1811, when

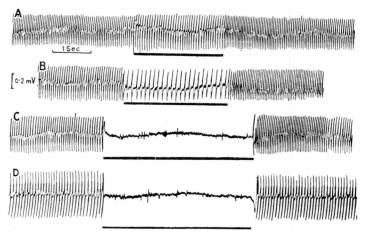

FIG. 66. OSCILLATING POTENTIALS OF THE SPINAL CORD OF A
DECEREBRATE AND CURARISED CAT

Recordings from a needle electrode in the anterior horn of a lumbar segment. *A, B* and *C:* stimulation of the anterior lobe of the cerebellum by increasing strengths of current. *D:* inhibition of the tetanus by stimulation of the caudally-directed inhibitory system found by Magoun in the brain stem.

(From Terzuolo (1954) *Arch. int. Physiol.*, **62**, 179.)

trying to puzzle out spinal reflexes, recognised that muscles had sensory as well as motor nerves which, he said, 'conveyed a sense of the condition of the muscles to the brain', and he spoke of a 'circle of nerves' making a sensory-motor junction between brain and muscle. What Bell called a circle of nerves we now call a feedback loop.

The main result of the actual demonstration of these feedback loops has been a greater understanding of sensory mechanisms and a revision of the age-long concept of a dichotomy consisting of a sensory system on the one hand, and a motor system on the other. The borderline between these neuronal mechanisms can no longer be so rigidly defined.

Oscillating Potentials of the Spinal Cord. That the spinal cord has apparently autonomous rhythmic electrical activity was first observed in frogs by Sechenov in 1881. In 1941 Bremer, working with cats, drew attention to the oscillating potentials recordable from the surface of the spinal cord and noted that they became markedly rhythmic following the intravenous injection of strychnine. Bremer regards these oscillations as a sign of auto-rhythmicity and has demonstrated that in strychnine tetanus they become synchronous throughout long stretches of cord. This synchrony can be maintained across a transection provided there is contact between the two cut surfaces. The synchronising influence would therefore seem to be exerted by an electrical field effect in this case.

Terzuolo found that these oscillatory potentials of strychnine tetanus (Fig. 66) are accelerated in frequency by stimulation of the caudally-directed facilitatory system found by Magoun in the brain stem, and cease abruptly on stimulation of the descending inhibitory system from the bulbar reticular formation (see Chapter 17). They are also influenced by cerebellar and vestibular stimulation mediated through the reticular formation. By extracellular recordings with microelectrodes, single units were found by Terzuolo and Gernandt to discharge in bursts that were coincident with the rising phase only of each wave of the oscillatory potentials. This fact, taken together with the demonstration by Fuortes and Frank of slow intracellular changes coincident with the tetanic oscillations, points to their reflecting fluctuations of membrane potential rather than envelopes of cell discharges. There is not at present evidence that defines whether these fluctuations take place at the membrane of the soma or of the dendrites. The problem is in many ways analogous to that of electroencephalographic potentials as discussed in Chapter 16.

BIBLIOGRAPHY

Barker, D. 'The Innervation of Mammalian Skeletal Muscle.' In *Myotatic, Kinesthetic and Vestibular Mechanisms. Ciba Symp.* (1967).

Barron, D. H. and Matthews, B. H. C. (1938) The interpretation of potential changes in the spinal cord. *J. Physiol. (Lond.)*, **92**, 276–321.

Barron, D. H. and Matthews, B. H. C. (1939) Dorsal root reflexes. *J. Physiol. (Lond.)*, **94**, 26–27 p.

Bernhard, C. F. (1953) 'Analysis of the Spinal Cord Potentials in Leads from the Cord Dorsum.' In *Ciba Foundation Symposium on the Spinal Cord*, Malcolm, J. (Ed.). Little, Brown, Boston.

Bonnet, V. and Bremer, F. (1938) Étude des potentiels électriques de la moelle épinière faisant suite chez le grenouille spinale à une ou deux volées d'influx centripètes. *C. R. Soc. Biol. (Paris)*, **127**, 806.

Boyd, I. S. (1962) The structure and innervation of the nuclear bag muscle fibre system and nuclear chain muscle fibre system in mammalian muscle. *Proc. roy. Soc. B.*, **245**, 81–136.

Bremer, F. (1941) Le tétanos strychnique et le méchanisme de la synchronisation neuronique. *Arch. int. Physiol.*, **51**, 211–260.

Brock, L. G., Coombs, J. S. and Eccles, J. C. (1952) The recording of potentials from motoneurones with an intracellular electrode. *J. Physiol. (Lond.)*, **117**, 431–460.

Eccles, J. C., Eccles, R. M. and Magni, F. (1961) Central inhibitory action attributable to presynaptic depolarisation produced by muscle afferent volleys. *J. Physiol. (Lond.)*, **159**, 147–166.

Eccles, J. C., Fatt, P. and Koketsu, K. (1954) Cholinergic and inhibitory synapses in a pathway from motor-axon collaterals to motoneurones. *J. Physiol. (Lond.)*, **126**, 524–562.

Eccles, J. C., Kostyuk, P. G. and Schmidt, R. F. (1962) The effect of electric polarisation of the spinal cord on central afferent fibres and on their excitatory synaptic action. *J. Physiol. (Lond.)*, **162**, 138–150.

Eccles, J. C., Kozak, W. and Magni, F. (1961) Dorsal root reflexes of muscle Group I afferent fibres. *J. Physiol. (Lond.)*, **159**, 128–146.

Eccles, J. C. and Krnjević, K. (1959) Presynaptic changes associated with post-tetanic potentiation in the spinal cord. *J. Physiol. (Lond.)*, **149**, 274–287.

Eccles, J. C., Schmidt, R. F. and Willis, W. D. (1962) Presynaptic inhibition of the spinal monosynaptic reflex pathway. *J. Physiol. (Lond.)*, **161**, 282–297.

Eccles, J. D., Schmidt, R. F. and Willis, W. D. (1963) Depolarisation of central terminals of Group Ib afferent fibres of muscle. *J. Neurophysiol.*, **26**, 1–27.

Eccles, J. C., Schmidt, R. F. and Willis, W. D. (1963) The location and the mode of action of the presynaptic inhibitory pathways on the Group I afferent fibres from muscle. *J. Neurophysiol.*, **26**, 506–522.

Eldred, E., Granit, R. and Merton, P. A. (1953) Supraspinal control of the muscle spindles and its significance. *J. Physiol. (Lond.)*, **122**, 498–523.

Forbes, A. (1922) Interpretation of spinal reflexes in terms of present knowledge of nerve conduction. *Physiol. Rev.*, **2**, 361–414.

Frank, K. and Fuortes, M. G. F. (1955) Potentials recorded from the spinal cord with microelectrodes. *J. Physiol. (Lond.)*, **130**, 625–654.

Frank, K. and Fuortes, M. G. F. (1956) Unitary activity of spinal interneurones of cats. *J. Physiol. (Lond.)*, **131**, 424–435.

Gasser, H. S. and Graham, H. T. (1933) Potentials produced in the spinal cord by stimulation of spinal roots. *Amer. J. Physiol.*, **103**, 303–320.

Granit, R. (1966) *Muscular Afferents and Motor Control*. Almquist and Wiksell, Stockholm, and Wiley, New York.

Hubbard, J. I. and Schmidt, R. F. (1963) An electrophysiological investigation of mammalian motor nerve terminals. *J. Physiol. (Lond.)*, **166**, 145–167.

Hunt, C. C. (1952) Muscle stretch receptors; peripheral mechanisms and reflex function. *Cold Spr. Harb. Symp. quant. Biol.*, **17**, 113–123.

Kuffler, S. W., Hunt, C. C. and Quilliam, J. P. (1951) Function of medullated small nerve fibers in mammalian ventral roots: efferent muscle spindle innervation. *J. Neurophysiol.*, **14**, 29–54.

Leksell, L. (1945) The action potential and excitatory effects of the small ventral root fibres to skeletal muscle. *Acta physiol. scand.*, **10**, Suppl. 31, 1–84.

Lloyd, D. P. C. (1941) A direct central inhibitory action of dromically conducted impulses. *J. Neurophysiol.*, **4**, 184–190.

Lloyd, D. P. C. (1943) Reflex action in relation to pattern and peripheral source of afferent stimulation. *J. Neurophysiol.*, **6**, 111–119.

Lloyd, D. P. C. (1943) Neuron patterns controlling transmission of ipsilateral hind limb reflexes in the cat. *J. Neurophysiol.*, **6**, 317–326.

Lloyd, D. P. C. (1946) Facilitation and inhibition of spinal motorneurons. *J. Neurophysiol.*, **9**, 421–438.

Lloyd, D. P. C. (1946) Integrative pattern of excitation and inhibition in two-neuron reflex arcs. *J. Neurophysiol.*, **9**, 439–444.

Lloyd, D. P. C. (1949) Post-tetanic potentiation of response in monosynaptic reflex pathways of the spinal cord. *J. gen. Physiol.*, **33**, 147–170.

Lloyd, D. P. C. (1951) Electrical signs of impulse conduction in spinal motoneurons. *J. gen. Physiol.*, **35**, 255–288.

Lloyd, D. P. C. (1951) After-currents, after-potentials, excitability, and ventral root electrotonus in spinal motoneurons. *J. gen. Physiol.*, **35**, 289–321.

Lloyd, D. P. C., Hunt, C. C. and McIntyre, A. K. (1955) Transmission in fractionated monosynaptic spinal reflex systems. *J. gen. Physiol.*, **38**, 307–317.

Lloyd, D. P. C. and McIntyre, A. K. (1949) On the origins of dorsal root potentials. *J. gen. Physiol.*, **32**, 409–443.

Renshaw, B. (1940) Activity in the simplest reflex pathways. *J. Neurophysiol.*, **3**, 373–387.

Renshaw, B. (1941) Influence of discharge of motoneurons upon excitation of neighboring motoneurons. *J. Neurophysiol.*, **4**, 167–183.

Renshaw, B. (1946) Central effects of centripetal impulses in axons of spinal ventral roots. *J. Neurophysiol.*, **9**, 191–204.

Scheibel, M. E. and Scheibel, A. B. (1966) Spinal motorneurones, interneurones and Renshaw cells. A Golgi study. *Arch. ital. Biol.*, **104**, 328–353.

Schmidt, R. F. and Willis, W. D. (1963) Depolarisation of central terminals of afferent fibres in the cervical spinal cord of the cat. *J. Neurophysiol.*, **26**, 44–60.

Sechenov, I. M. (1881) Galvanische Erscheinungen an der cerebro-spinalen Axe des Frosches. *Pflüger's Arch. ges. Physiol.*, **25**, 281–284.

Sherrington, C. S. (1947) *Integrative Action of the Nervous System*, 2nd ed. Cambridge University Press, London.

Terzuolo, C. and Gernandt, B. E. (1956) Spinal unit activity during synchronisation of a convulsive type (strychnine tetanus). *Amer. J. Physiol.*, **186**, 263–270.

Wall, P. D. (1958) Excitability changes in afferent fibre terminations and their relation to slow potentials. *J. Physiol. (Lond.)*, **142**, 1–21.

Woodbury, J. W. and Patton, H. D. (1954) Electrical activity of single spinal cord elements. *Cold Spr. Harb. Symp. quant. Biol.*, **17**, 185–188.

The Electrical Response to Stimulation of Sense Organs

THE child in the nursery is taught that he has five senses, but in fact he has so many more that a physiologist would hesitate to put a number to them. The senses of muscle movement, of pain, of balance and of temperature are some of the important ones omitted from the usual categories of sight, hearing, smell, touch, and taste. The sense organs are man's only source of information about his environment, and his only clue to a change in this environment is a change in one or more of these organs.

The modern development of electron microscopy has added greatly to our knowledge of the morphology of the various endings and the intricacies of their innervation, and the successful exploitation of microelectrode recording from the receptors themselves is beginning to relate structure and function.

Each sense has its own end-organ, grading in complexity from the simplest form of the free nerve-ending to the intricate structure in the retina of the eye. Some of these end-organs are specific to a single type of stimulus; for example, Meissner corpuscles, the encapsulated receptors in the skin, respond to touch but do not signal pain. But the specificity of reaction ends at the sense-organ; the messages carried from them in the nerves running to the central nervous system are all alike, all are the familiar action potential of the nerve fibre, specificity of sensation depending on where in the brain these impulses arrive. One of the first proofs that stimulation of an end-organ produces action potentials in its sensory nerve came from the experiments of Forbes on muscle stretching, which were also some of the earliest experiments in which valve amplification was applied to electrophysiology. The type of impression received by the brain from these showers of action spikes is dependent on the topographical pattern of the fibres conveying them, the relative frequency of discharge in each component fibre and the temporal patterning of this discharge in each fibre. Some sense endings, unlike the muscle spindles which respond to stretch, share nerve fibres; for example, there may be as many as four Pacinian corpuscles (the specific pressure receptors) served by the branches of the same sensory fibre. The sensation experienced must clearly be influenced by this sharing of innervation.

Given a definite pattern and frequency, travelling from the periphery in a set of afferent fibres the message will be the same whether this pattern has been set up at the receptor or artificially somewhere along the nerve fibre. If one bumps one's elbow, the ulnar nerve signals a message from the little finger although this was not involved in the original injury which took place on the nerve path between the finger and the central nervous system.

Volta carried out many experiments on himself to find out the effect of an electric current on the organs of sense. He gave a vivid description of his sensations in a letter written in his quaint French to Sir Joseph Banks in 1800. He describes the tingling in his fingers caused by applied currents and the very great increase in sensation at the site of a cut ('une douleur si vive et si cuisante'). He also describes the sensation of a sharp taste when current was applied to the tip of the tongue, the sensation of light when it was passed through his eyeballs, and, when applied to his ears, the strangest of sounds, like the bubbling of a thick paste ('comme si quelque pâte ou matière tenace bouillonoit'). He failed to produce a sensation of smell in his nose. He also speaks of the shock he felt in his brain when he passed the current through his head and expresses the fear that it may be dangerous to repeat this experience very often, a piece of advice now frequently neglected.

Several attempts have been made to formulate a law relating degrees of sensation to intensity of stimulation. The most famous of these is the Weber-Fechner Law which states that sensation is proportional to the logarithm of the stimulus, or more exactly, that sensation $= K \log I + C$, where I is the intensity of the stimulus, and K and C are constants. The concept of such a law raised a storm in the middle of the last century because Fechner, who besides being a physicist was a religious mystic, a poet, and above all a Romantic, tended to regard it as the expression of the relationship between the body and the mind, between man's environment and his 'psyche'. It is, of course, no longer regarded with such mysticism since all it demonstrates (and that not too well) is the relationship between the stimulus and the event at the distant end of a nerve pathway.

The law has been greatly criticised, even in its more material interpretation, since it does not hold for the senses of taste or smell and holds only within a limited range for sight and pressure. One reason for this has been analysed by Hoagland, who has shown that for many senses the Weber-Fechner Law represents the mid-region of an integral distribution curve; such a curve is to be expected from the addition, with increasing intensity of stimulus, of more and more active receptors. The law, originally intended to describe intensity, most nearly holds for pitch discrimination.

As we have already seen, a nerve, when stimulated by a direct current, does not continue to respond because the fibre becomes adapted to the unchanging quality of the stimulus (see page 85). A less immediate form of adaptation is seen in sense-organs where it has importance in relation to the function of the particular end-organ concerned. In frog's muscle spindles, for example, the nerve's response to a constant stretching of the muscle, as Matthews and Adrian showed, is a shower of action spikes falling off in frequency as the stretch is prolonged. The decline in frequency of the response of a nerve after a load of 2 g had been hung from the tendon of the muscle is graphed in Fig. 67, taken from Matthews. This falling off, or adaptation rate, is more rapid with a severe stretch than with a weak stretch; in other words, the high impulse-frequency induced by a strong stimulus declines more rapidly than the slower discharge of a less intense stimulus. Thus the end-organ's power to set up nerve impulses is impaired not only by the length of time it has been stimulated but also by the intensity of the stimulus applied.

Muscle spindles, however, are, compared with other end-organs, slow to adapt, and respond to a constant stimulus with a comparatively long-persisting series of discharges. This makes them useful recorders of limb position, since were they to adapt quickly, the organism would rapidly lose its source of information as to body posture.

Some end-organs are more rapidly adapting as, for example, hair and touch receptors. These respond to a constant stimulus with only one or two discharges and then cease to register another response unless a change of stimulus occurs. This is, perhaps, as well for man, since he has evolved a pattern of

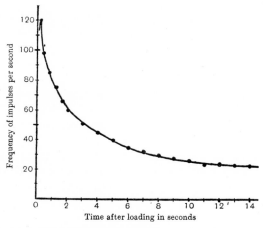

FIG. 67. THE DECLINE IN FREQUENCY OF THE RESPONSE IN THE NERVE AFTER A LOAD OF 2 g IS HUNG ON THE THREAD FROM THE TENDON

Frog's nerve: temperature 15°C.
(From Matthews (1931) *J. Physiol.* (*Lond.*), **71**, 64.)

society which demands that the tactile receptors in his skin receive the continuous stimuli of clothes. In the Oxford laboratories, however, a second type of tactile receptor, which is slow in adapting, has been found in the skin.

Another example of slowly-adapting end-organs is found in the carotid sinus. The carotid sinus is an area of widening in the internal carotid artery in which there are two types of endorgan, one sensitive to chemical changes in blood composition and concerned with control of respiration, and the other responding to blood pressure changes within the sinus. The impulses set up by these pressure endings were studied by Bronk in single fibres of the carotid sinus nerve, and were found to adapt more slowly than any other end-organ yet studied. This can be seen in Fig. 68, which illustrates the steady rhythmic discharge at four different levels of pressure in the carotid sinus. At none of these pressures is there any sign of adaptation, but the increasing frequency of discharge with

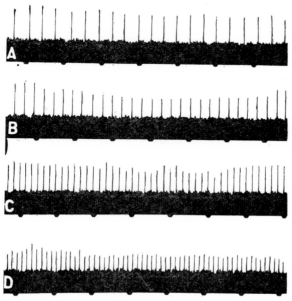

FIG. 68. AFFERENT IMPULSES FROM A SINGLE END-ORGAN IN THE CAROTID SINUS STIMULATED BY CONSTANT PRESSURES WITHIN THE SINUS

A, 40 mm Hg; *B,* 80 mm Hg; *C,* 140 mm Hg; *D,* 200 mm Hg. Time marker: 1/5 sec.

(From Bronk and Stella (1935) *Amer. J. Physiol.,* **110,** 708.)

rising pressure is very marked. Since these receptors are the initiators of the reflex which controls blood pressure their efficiency is clearly enhanced by this slowness of adaptation, for it enables them to remain responsive to mean blood pressure in spite of the intermittent stimuli of systole and diastole. Other slowly adapting end-organs are found in the stretch receptors of the lung. These, whose fibres are part of the vagus nerve, respond to inflation of the lung and are quiescent during expiration, as can be seen in Fig. 69. These impulses form the first station on a reflex path controlling respiratory movements (although this is not the sole mechanism initiating action of respiratory muscles). The nerve is actually more speedily adapting than any end-organ for it may respond to a weak constant current with but a single impulse, and even to a strong current with only a short burst of impulses.

The characteristics of adaptation in nerve and in end-organs are strikingly different from fatigue on many counts. In the first place, the time relations are quite different; not only does adaptation develop more quickly than fatigue but recovery from it is almost instantaneous on removal of the stimulus,

FIG. 69. RHYTHMIC GROUPS OF IMPULSES IN A SINGLE MOTOR NERVE FIBRE TO AN EXTERNAL INTERCOSTAL MUSCLE IN THE CAT

Time marker: 1/5 sec. Lower line: pneumogram, upward movement indicating inspiration.

(From Bronk and Ferguson (1935) *Amer. J. Physiol.*, **110**, 700.)

instead of taking many minutes. Another outstanding difference is in the response to anoxia: fatigue in nerve is greatly hastened by lack of oxygen supply whereas adaptation is scarcely affected even when pure nitrogen is substituted for air. Adaptation clearly cannot be as directly dependent on oxidative processes as is recovery in nerve.

Perhaps the most striking distinction between the behaviour of adapted nerve and fatigued nerve is the ability, alluded to above, of the former to respond instantly to an increase in intensity of stimulus. A nerve which has adapted to a state of complete unresponsiveness to a constant stimulus will react to a sudden increase in the strength of the stimulus, thus demonstrating that its excitability is preserved. A nerve fatigued to unresponsiveness cannot be excited by any change in intensity of stimulation. That end-organs show the same property of adaptation has been proved by Adrian for the pressure receptors of the cat's toe pad.

These findings make it only reasonable to postulate a similar mechanism for adaptation in the end-organ and in the nerve.

In line with the classical membrane theory of nervous conduction outlined in a previous section this would regard adaptation as another example of surface depolarisation, a disturbance of the surface charge which prevents the building up of impulse discharges at the maximal rate. Matthews demonstrated the influence of ions on the response of muscle spindles to stretch; reduction of calcium in the surrounding fluid increases the rate of adaptation in receptors and so does an increase in potassium. It has been postulated that depolarisation results from disintegration of the surface layers by deformation caused by the mechanical stress. Cattell and Hoagland carried this study further in work with the tactile receptors in frogs' skin, experiments which gave support to the surmise that the important ion is potassium. The adaptation of these cutaneous sensory endings in the frog is accompanied by the accumulation of K ions, although this is not universally the case for all sensory endings. An alternative theory of adaptation in nerve is that the constantly-applied stimulus sets up an opposing reaction tending to stabilise the fibre; this derives from the hypothesis of Lorente de Nó outlined in Chapter 8.

The tendency of some types of invertebrate axons to respond repetitively to stimulation by weak direct currents has been the subject of extensive studies (Fessard, Arvanitaki, Skoglund, Hodgkin). Although this is essentially a property of unmyelinated nerve and is seen at its best in crustacean nerve, the analogy to the response of some sensory organs is marked, as can be seen by comparing Fig. 70 with Fig. 68, which records the response of a slowly-adapting sense organ to a constant stimulus. In both these cases (each of which records the response of single units) there is increase in frequency of discharge with increasing intensity, but no decrease in spike height with persisting stimulation. Hodgkin and Arvanitaki have both found other types of crustacean fibre whose action potentials fall off in frequency though not in spike height with continued stimulation by direct currents; these records are strikingly similar to those of Adrian and others on the more rapidly-adapting sense organs such as touch receptors, and it is inevitable that one should wonder whether the unmyelinated terminal fibres of some sensory nerves may not perhaps share this property of repetitive response.

The type of impulse carried by the sensory fibre is the same whatever its source of origin, and the final discrimination as to the locale of this origin must depend on the central connexions of the specific fibres carrying messages. These fibres are very highly specific to the sense organs they serve. For example, working with the thermal receptors of the cat's tongue, Zotterman has found the differentiation between increase and

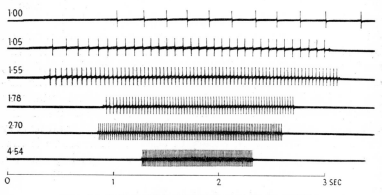

FIG. 70. REPETITIVE RESPONSES IN CRAB NERVE

Electrical changes at the stimulating electrode produced by sudden application of constant currents with strengths shown relative to the rheobase. The beginning and end of the applied current is marked by the slight artefact.

(From Hodgkin (1948) *J. Physiol. (Lond.)*, **107**, 165.)

decrease in temperature to be based on a peripheral specialisation of afferent fibre and, by inference, of receptor. As can be seen from Fig. 71, rise in temperature from 25° to 40°C was signalled by a burst of discharges in the fibre from a warmth receptor and electrical silence in that from the cold receptor. When the temperature fell, this change evoked a shower of high-frequency discharges in the previously quiescent 'cold' fibre. This simple relation does not hold for all conditions of temperature change and many have been shown by Zotterman and his colleagues to be of considerable complexity. Recordings, like these, from the afferent nerve tell us only about the form of the message as it travels from the periphery and no knowledge is yet available about the mechanism by which thermal receptors are excited or how they initiate these nerve impulses.

Temperature mechanisms such as have just been discussed refer only to surface receptors and the messages they send to the brain. Overall regulation of body temperature is controlled by the anterior hypothalamus which contains thermally-sensitive neurones that have been demonstrated by Magoun and his collaborators to initiate heat loss by panting, sweating and rapid respiration. The local electrical sign of this central response to heat is a slow potential change, found by von Euler

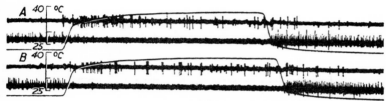

FIG. 71. SIMULTANEOUS MICROELECTRODE RECORDINGS FROM A 'WARMTH' FIBRE FROM THE CHORDA TYMPANI (IN THE UPPER TRACE) AND FROM A 'COLD' FIBRE FROM THE LINGUAL NERVE BELOW (CAT)

Rise in temperature causes activity in the former and electrical silence in the latter. Fall in temperature has the opposite effect.

(From Dodt and Zotterman (1952) *Acta physiol. scand.*, **26**, 345.)

to vary by about $\frac{1}{2}$ to 1 mV for every 1/10th degree centigrade change of temperature in the anterior hypothalamus.

The mechanism by which a sense organ initiates a nerve impulse in a sensory nerve has been most fully explored in the stretch receptor in muscle. Kuffler and Eyzaguirre with intra-cellular electrodes in single sensory neurones of the stretch receptor of the crayfish have shown the precipitating cause to be distortion of the dendrites by the movement of the muscle strands in which their terminals lie. Stretching produces a proportional depolarisation of the dendrites which spreads electrotonically to the cell body whose resting potential is there-by reduced, also in a graded fashion. If this reduction of soma potential reaches a certain threshold a propagated action potential is fired down the axon. In this case, then, it is the dendritic membrane that is the transducer of mechanical to electrical activity.

The stretch receptor of the lobster is a particularly interesting

sense organ for it has been found by Kuffler to have two inhibitory fibres synapsing on to the dendrites of a single afferent
neurone. These two inhibitory fibres have different properties,
as can be seen from Fig. 72. The action of these fibres seems
to be a controlling one in that they act to repolarise the membrane of the sensory neurone. Kuffler has found no evidence
that this restoration of charge on the membrane reaches a
stage of hyperpolarisation. Peripheral inhibitory neurones,

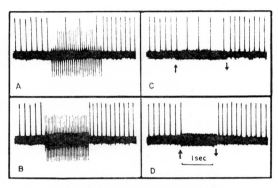

FIG. 72. TWO TYPES OF INHIBITORY FIBRE ACTING ON A SINGLE
STRETCH RECEPTOR OF THE LOBSTER

Left: One of these fibres if stimulated at 15/sec only partially inhibits discharge from the receptor (*A*). At 20/sec inhibition is complete (*B*).
Right: The other fibre requires stimulation at 30/sec to produce partial
inhibition (*C*), and at 40/sec to make this complete (*D*). Period of inhibitor
stimulation in *A* and *B* marked by artefacts, in *C* and *D* by arrows.

(From Kuffler (1957) *Nature*, **180**, 1490.)

however, have been found only in invertebrates, the only
known inhibitory mechanism in vertebrate animals being
entirely within central nervous system structures.

Another type of sense ending that is activated mechanically
is the Pacinian corpuscle, the pressure receptor that has been
the subject of special study by Gray and his associates. Their
findings in the cat have led them to the opinion that the initiating event is a change in the membrane of the terminal portion
of the sensory fibre that lies inside the receptor capsule (though
whether this change is caused by distortion or by compression
is not yet known). The membrane of these non-myelinated
fibre endings has specialised properties in that pressure on

the Pacinian corpuscle evokes a graded potential proportional to the amplitude and rate of change of mechanical deformation (Fig. 73). This summating potential in the terminals spreads electrotonically along the fibre, reaching the first node of Ranvier (which also lies within the capsule of the receptor) and when a critical level of potential has been amassed at this

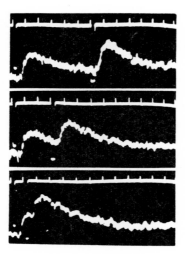

FIG. 73. SUMMATION OF RECEPTOR POTENTIALS WITH DIFFERENT INTERVALS BETWEEN STIMULI. PACINIAN CORPUSCLE

Upper traces: Time in msec. Breaks indicate occurrence of stimulus.
Lower traces: Summating receptor potentials.
(From Gray and Sato (1953) *J. Physiol. (Lond.)*, **122**, 610.)

point an all-or-nothing spike potential is triggered at the node and propagated up the fibre.

The first node of Ranvier lies within the corpuscle and was earlier thought to be the sole site of action potential initiation. More recent work, however, has shown that the unmyelinated nerve terminals are also capable of spike genesis.

The receptors are, therefore, transducers converting various forms of energy into electricity; this change takes place in the receptor itself setting up a generator potential.

Generator potentials have been recorded directly from Pacinian corpuscles, from the stretch receptor of the crayfish and from the mammalian muscle spindles. Because the generator potential is a graded one it may be said that the rate of discharge in the sensory nerve reflects the strength of the stimulus, though it would be more accurate to say that the rate of rise in amplitude of the summating generator potential is the determinant of the initial discharge frequency of the action potentials that carry the message to the central nervous system and these are, therefore, initially dependent on the rate of depolarisation of the receptor membrane.

As described above, the relationship between intensity and frequency is lost when adaptation occurs, for the rate of discharge in the afferent nerve declines—this in itself being directly caused by decrease in rate of the generator potential. The mechanism of this adaptive process within the receptor is the subject of much current research.

One of the outstanding developments of modern neurophysiology has been the recognition of control by the brain over sensory inflow from the receptors and the discovery of the neural pathways through which some of these mechanisms operate. Reference has already been made to the fine fibre control of stretch receptors in muscle (see page 129), and in later chapters some discussion will be found of evidence that has accumulated for analogous centrifugal control in the auditory, visual and olfactory systems. This is a type of control exercised over the information that is allowed to proceed from the receptor into the central nervous system, rather than a control introduced at a higher level of integration. Many types of central control, by facilitation and inhibition of output of motor nerve impulses, have been known for some time (see, for example, Chapter 9). This more recently acquired knowledge of control over input of sensory impulses begins to fill out the picture of integration of sensory experience and to suggest ways in which the central nervous system handles the mechanisms for editing sensory impressions so that some receive attention at the expense of others.

BIBLIOGRAPHY

Adrian, E. D. (1928) *The Basis of Sensation.* Christophers, London.
Adrian, E. D. (1947) *The Physical Background of Perception.* Clarendon Press, Oxford.

Adrian, E. D. (1949) *Sensory Integration. 1st Sherrington Lecture.* University Press, Liverpool.

Arvanitaki, A. (1938) 'Les variations graduées de la polarisation des systèmes excitables.' In *Physiologie Générale du Système Nerveux.* Hermann, Paris.

Burgen, A. S. V. and Kuffler, S. W. (1957) Two inhibitory fibres forming synapses with a single nerve cell in the lobster. *Nature,* **180,** 1490–1491.

Davis, H. (1961) Some principles of sensory receptor action. *Physiol. Rev.,* **41,** 391–416.

Diamond, J., Gray, J. A. B. and Sato, M. (1956) The site of initiation of impulses in Pacinian corpuscles. *J. Physiol. (Lond.),* **133,** 54–57.

Dodt, E. and Zotterman, Y. (1952) Mode of action of warm receptors. *Acta physiol. scand.,* **26,** 345–377.

Fechner, G. T. (1862) *Elemente der Psychophysik.* Breitkopf and Hartel, Leipzig.

Fessard, A. (1936) *Propriétés Rythmiques de la Matière Vivante.* Hermann, Paris.

Forbes, A., Campbell, C. J. and Williams, H. B. (1924) Electrical records of afferent nerve impulses from muscular receptors. *Amer. J. Physiol.,* **69,** 283–303.

Granit, R. (1955) *Receptors and Sensory Perception.* Yale University Press, New Haven.

Gray, J. A. B. and Sato, M. (1953) Properties of the receptor potential in Pacinian corpuscles. *J. Physiol. (Lond.),* **122,** 610–636.

Gray, J. A. B. (1959) Mechanical into electrical energy in certain mechanoreceptors. *Progr. Biophys.,* **9,** 286–324.

Hodgkin, A. L. (1948) Repetitive action in nerve. *J. Physiol. (Lond.),* **107,** 165–181.

Hunt, C. C. and Takeuchi, A. (1962) Responses of the nerve terminal of the Pacinian corpuscle. *J. Physiol. (Lond.),* **160,** 1–21.

Iggo, A. (1960) Cutaneous mechanoreceptors with afferent C-fibres. *J. Physiol. (Lond.),* **152,** 337–353.

Katz, B. (1950) Depolarisation of sensory terminals and the initiation of impulses in the muscle spindle. *J. Physiol.,* **111,** 261–282.

Kuffler, S. W. and Eyzaguirre, C. (1955) Synaptic inhibition in an isolated nerve cell. *J. gen. Physiol.,* **39,** 155–184.

Lowenstein, W. R. and Rathkamp, R. (1958) The sites for mechanicoelectric conversion in a Pacinian corpuscle. *J. gen. Physiol.,* **41,** 1245–1265.

Matthews, B. H. C. (1931) The response of a muscle spindle during active contraction of a muscle. *J. Physiol. (Lond.),* **72,** 153–174.

Mendelson, M. and Lowenstein, W. R. (1964) Mechanisms of receptor adaptation. *Science*, **144**, 554–555.

Ozeki, M. and Sato, M. (1964) Initiation of impulses at the non-myelinated nerve terminals in Pacinian corpuscles. *J. Physiol. (Lond.)*, **170**, 167–185.

Pease, D. C. and Quilliam, T. A. (1957) Electron microscopy of the Pacinian corpuscle. *J. biophys. biochem. Cytol.*, **3**, 331–342.

Terzuolo, C. A. and Washizu, Y. (1962) Relation between stimulus strength, generator potential and impulse frequency in stretch receptor of crustacea. *J. Neurophysiol.*, **25**, 56–66.

Weddell, G. (1961) 'Receptors for Somatic Sensation.' In *Brain and Behavior*. Brazier, M. A. B. (Ed.) Vol. 2. American Institute of Biological Science, Washington.

Zotterman, Y. (1954) 'Sensory Receptors.' In *Transactions of the 4th Conference on the Nerve Impulse*. Nachmansohn, D. (Ed.). Josiah Macy r. Foundation, New York.

The Electrical Activity of the Auditory System

In 1930 two workers at Princeton startled physiologists with an experiment on a cat in which they demonstrated that by placing electrodes on the auditory nerve they could, with amplification, hear in the next room the sounds falling on the cat's ear. These sounds were so exactly reproduced that not only the words but the voice of the speaker could be identified. They at first concluded that the impulses in the nerve reproduced faithfully the frequencies of the sound waves. Their experimental findings, which is named after them the 'Wever-Bray effect', has been confirmed by many other observers, but on further work they found their original interpretation could not be maintained. Even at face value there are many details which elude such an explanation. For example, there is the fact that frequencies as high as 70,000 c/s can be followed in the cat and even higher (100,000) in some bats, a rate which would impose on the auditory nerve a refractory period far shorter than the shortest known; also these responses neither follow the all-or-nothing law, nor do they show the usual form of fatigue; finally, they persist not only during anaesthesia but also for some time after death. This effectively excludes the nerve impulse as a factor in their conduction.

It is now established beyond doubt that the sounds heard are the microphonic response of the cochlea, a mechanical effect of the wave of pressure directly transformed into an electrical signal. This signal is unlike a nerve-action potential; the action potential is always negative, but the microphonic response follows the polarity of the stimulating pulse and reverses with it.

The microphonic potential may reach an amplitude of one mV and follows with very short latency and with extreme faithfulness the wave-form of the auditory stimulus, as well as its intensity. It can be recorded not only from the nerve but from any tissue near to the cochlea, and especially well from the round window. The nature of this microphonic response will become clearer when the structure of the ear has been briefly reviewed.

The sound waves are funnelled by the auricle into the external auditory canal where they impinge on the eardrum, or tympanic membrane, which in the normal ear completely

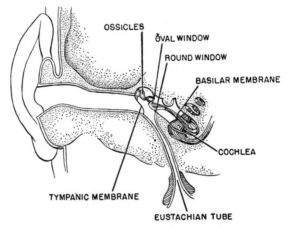

FIG. 74. GENERAL STRUCTURE OF THE EAR IN MAN

closes off the end of this canal. On the other side of this membrane is the middle ear, a cavity filled with air and, during yawning or swallowing, open to atmospheric pressure by way of the eustachian tube leading to the nasopharynx. In mammals the inner surface of the eardrum has a bony articulating connexion through three ossicles (the malleus, the incus and the stapes) to the oval window, one of the two openings in the temporal bone which divides the middle from the inner-ear cavity. The second opening in the temporal bone is covered by the membrane of the round window and it is here, at these two windows, that the sound-wave ceases to be airborne and becomes fluid-borne by the perilymph which fills the inner ear. Within the inner ear lies the organ of hearing, the cochlea. These several structures can be identified in the diagram of the internal ear shown in Fig. 74.

Two pathways for the sound-wave to the fluid surrounding the cochlea have been indicated: a mechanical movement of the ossicles against the oval window (which is the principal route), and an airborne wave vibrating the membrane of the round window. There is yet a third, which is by direct bone conduction through the skull, a pathway utilised by hearing aids for deafness due to blockage of air-conducted sound in the middle ear.

The cochlea is a spiral passage winding into the bone of the skull; in man it takes the form of a canal about 3 cm long,

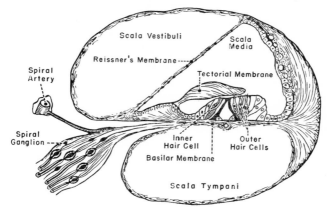

FIG. 75. CROSS-SECTION OF THE COCHLEAR CANAL
(After Rasmussen (1947) *Some Trends in Neuroanatomy*. Brown, Dubuque.)

coiling like a snail shell $2\frac{3}{4}$ times round a conical core. This canal is divided along its length, the partition being partly by a bony shelf and partly by a strong membrane. This membrane plays an essential role in the function of hearing, since it is on the inner surface of this, the basilar membrane, that the organ of Corti lies. The ultimate sense-endings for hearing are the hair cells which are found in the organ of Corti; these are each directly innervated by multiple fibres of the bipolar nerve cells in the spiral ganglion whose axons pass in the acoustic branch of the eighth nerve to the cochlear nucleus in the medulla.

An important feature of the cochlear structure, which is shown in Fig. 75, is the division of the canal into tunnels; two of these, the scala vestibuli and the scala tympani, are filled with perilymph (which resembles cerebrospinal fluid in composition) and are connected only by a small channel at the tip of the cochlea, in the apex of the spiral. The third tunnel, the scala media, contains endolymph (of very different ionic composition) and has no opening into either the scala vestibuli or the scala tympani.

A sound wave vibrates the eardrum, rocks the ossicles and causes changes in pressure on the oval window; these pressure changes are communicated directly to the fluid in the tunnel above the basilar membrane. A positive pressure in this tunnel, the scala media, distorts the basilar membrane downwards increasing the pressure in the scala tympani and bulges the round window outwards; conversely a negative pressure draws the basilar membrane upward; the alternation of pressure in acoustic waves makes the membrane vibrate.

There is a large standing potential difference of the scala media relative to the scala vestibuli and scala tympani. This is known as the endocochlear potential, the scala media being positive by about 80 mV to the other two. This potential difference is modulated by movement of the membranes enclosing the scala media when pressure is exerted on the oval window by sound; when tones are used as the stimulus, a graded 'summating potential' has been found by Davis to follow the envelope of the tone. The endocochlear potential is exquisitely sensitive to changes in oxygen supply, implying a dependence on metabolic rather than neuronal activity. Davis has suggested that the standing potential may serve an accessory function in the overall mechanism of hearing—namely to hyperpolarise the hair cells and thereby increase their sensitivity.

The microphonic action of the cochlea is undoubtedly a delicate mechanism for transforming mechanical force into electrical energy, but whether or not the cochlear microphonics are the element responsible for initiating impulses in the acoustic nerve has been for years one of the major controversies in the field of audition.

There have been many theories as to the actual stimulus from the hair cell that sets up an impulse in the nerve; the latency of the action potential response (about 0·6 msec) gave support to the school that at one time held the stimulus to be a chemical substance released by the hair cell when distorted, though the data do not necessarily impose this interpretation. The terminal fibres of the auditory nerve are very fine and consequently have a low conduction velocity.

Tasaki was the first to succeed (in 1954) in recording from the single fibres of the auditory nerve, and his observations have led him to the opinion that the mechanism of stimulation of the nerve is the current of the microphonic potential flowing through the hair cells from the scala vestibuli to the scala media. Whatever the nature of the initial stimulus, the end-organs so stimulated evoke action potentials which conform in every way to those found in other nerves of the body. They give an all-or-nothing response, have a refractory period, and signal change in intensity by change in frequency of discharge.

The response recordable at the cochlea is, therefore, a dual effect: the mechanical vibration causes the microphonic potential of Wever and Bray, while the action potential set up in the sensory pathways is the true auditory response. Figure 76 shows these two types of response to a single brief click as recorded by Rosenblith from the round window in a cat's ear.

In Fig. 76, the records a, b, d, e were obtained by means of a gross wire electrode located on the bone close to the round window membrane with the second on a remote inactive place.

In record a the most prominent components of the complex pattern that makes up the cochlear response are identified. A is the artefact indicating the occurrence of the electrical click. M is the earliest and most prominent component of the round-window response. It is exclusively the cochlear microphonic response of the hair cells. N_1 and N_2 are the most striking neural components that occur in round window records. N_1 is the response of the auditory nerve and N_2 a mixture of multiple elements of the primary neurone discharge with action potentials of the secondary neurones in the cochlear nucleus.

Record a represents the cochlear response to a click that is about 45 db above the threshold for hearing in man. Record b is for a click about 25 db above the threshold for man. A comparison of b with a shows the differential decrease in response for microphonic and neural components. The greater latency for N_1 and N_2 when compared with figure a is also noticeable.

Records *d* and *e* (both taken for clicks that lie about 40 db above the threshold for hearing in man) illustrate the contrast between microphonic and neural components in a different

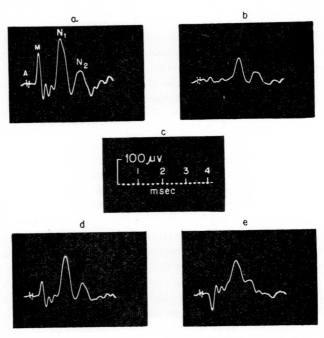

FIG. 76. THE MICROPHONIC RESPONSE (M) AND THE NERVE
RESPONSES (N₁ AND N₂) RECORDED AT THE ROUND WINDOW IN A
CAT'S EAR (PENTOBARBITAL ANAESTHESIA)

Record *a* at 45 db, record *b* at 25 db above human threshold. Records *d* and *e* illustrate the reversal of polarity in the microphonic response but not in the neural response. Negativity is recorded in an upward direction. *c* gives the time and voltage scales for the four records. See text.
(*Recording by courtesy of W. Rosenblith*)

manner. In *d* and *e* the stimulus is the same except that the polarity of its current has been reversed in *e*. Notice that *M*, the potential wave that represents the microphonic action of the cochlea, follows this reversal in polarity while N_1 and N_2 do not.

The range of frequency perceptible to normal human hearing is much greater than it is usually called upon to cover; the ear

can detect frequencies from about 20 c/s to between 20,000 and
30,000 (and higher still by bone conduction), but is most
sensitive to frequencies between 1,000 and 3,000 c/s, the most
important range for intelligibility of the human voice. These
limits far exceed the range in common use. The ultrasonic
note of the flying bat has a frequency of about 100,000 to
50,000 c/s (a range inaudible to man) emitted by the animal
in short spurts lasting a few thousandths of a second with
silent intervals. It is the mechanical production of this repetitive break in the singing note, which can be heard by the
human ear.

The crude differential response to frequency is, as Helmholtz
deduced, made by the end-organ, but the finer discrimination of
pitch takes place more centrally. Békésy's mechanical measurements have shown that the spiral design of the cochlea is such
that the basilar membrane responds maximally at different frequencies in different parts of the helix; the base vibrating
most to the higher frequencies and the apex to the lower, with a
progressive gradation between them. However, only at levels
of low intensity is the differentiation of area sharp; as the
intensity of the tone rises, wider and wider areas of the basilar
membrane are set in motion.

Tasaki's direct recordings from fibres of the auditory nerve
are in keeping with a spatial correlate of frequency being
activated at the cochlear nucleus, though not of the kind that
had been conjectured by previous workers. All the fibres he
recorded from were activated by a broad band of tones but
were differentiated by their level of cut-off at the high-frequency
end. This cut-off was found to be quite abrupt for any specific
fibre. Hence from Tasaki's findings, it would seem that the
number of activated fibres and their spatial distribution within
the cochlear nucleus is what signals to this first relay station
the frequency of the initiating tone, the higher the tone the
fewer the presynaptic fibres active at the mosaic of synapses in
the nucleus.

A mechanism for the further sharpening of pitch discrimination has been revealed by Galambos's demonstration that a
given tone may activate some units in the cochlear nucleus
while inhibiting others. Yet others may be unaffected by that
tone, hence the spatial patterning of activated, inhibited and

unaffected units may be specific for each tone in the audible frequency range.

Like other sensory responses, the auditory one with increasing intensity of stimulus shows an increase in rate of discharge in each unit as well as a recruitment of other units. For each frequency there are many units that can respond and they are recruited successively as the intensity is raised (i.e. as larger areas of the basilar membrane vibrate). The discharges in these neurones also show adaptation to a constant stimulus, the frequency of the action spikes falling off as the sound persists.

The second-order neurones of the dorsal cochlear nucleus cross to the superior olive of the opposite side where many terminate. In the monkey (though not in the cat) a few fibres after crossing ascend without synapsing to the medial geniculate body. The majority of the third-order neurones in the superior olive send their axons via the lateral lemniscus to the inferior colliculus where some cross to the opposite side. Again there is a species difference as to how many of these synapse on their way in the nucleus of the lateral lemniscus. No crossed pathway exists at the thalamic level. Some afferents from the ventral cochlear nucleus enter the superior olive of the same side so that each ear is already bilaterally represented at this level of the brain stem. The fourth-order neurones in the medial geniculate pass in the auditory radiations to the auditory cortex.

Important collateral pathways from the lateral lemniscus to the cerebellum were identified (electrophysiologically) by Snider and Stowell, and fibres from the dorsal cochlear nucleus to the reticular formation in the monkey were traced (anatomically) by Barnes, Magoun and Ranson. The schema of the ascending pathways shown on the left of Fig. 77 is adapted from the figure compiled by Davis from the data of the latter two groups of investigators together with that of Ades and the classical contributions of Ramón y Cajal.

Both Held and Ramón y Cajal, in the last century, identified collaterals from the main auditory pathway passing into the reticular formation of the brain stem. The anatomical existence of such collaterals has been confirmed by many subsequent investigators (notably by Winkler; by Barnes and collaborators; by Rasmussen; and by Stotler). Only in recent years has some light been shed on the functional role of these collaterals. This has come from the work of Magoun and his group on the ascending activating system of the brain stem (see Chapter 17) and their demonstration by electrophysiological techniques of

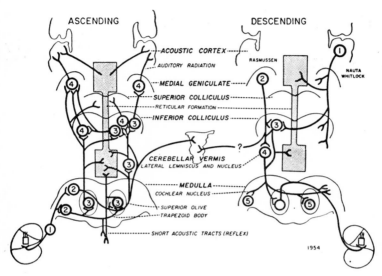

FIG. 77.

On left: The afferent auditory pathways. Second, third and fourth order neurones are indicated by numerals.
On right: The descending pathways of the auditory system.
(From Galambos (1956) *Ann. Otol. (St Louis)*, **65**, 1053.)

a pathway to the cortex that bypasses the specific relay nuclei of the thalamus.

In the classical route from the cochlear to the cortex the latency of response to a loud sound (in the cat) is about 8 msec at the auditory cortex, though it increases as the intensity of the stimulus drops. In the reticular core there is some topographical arrangement, for latencies in this non-specific system vary in some degree with locus, though as French and his collaborators have shown, they are in all cases longer than in the specific system and the responses are more diffusely distributed in the cortex. A slowly, as well as a rapidly-conducting system of ascending auditory connexions had been postulated ten years earlier on purely anatomical grounds by Barnes, Magoun and Ranson.

In Fig. 78 are records of the response of the cat's auditory cortex to a brief click; the first phase of the response is surface positive, the second surface negative.

In the unanaesthetised animal the later response that has ascended via the reticular core of the brain stem can also be recorded. That this system is not dependent on the integrity of the specific auditory pathways is shown by the fact that when

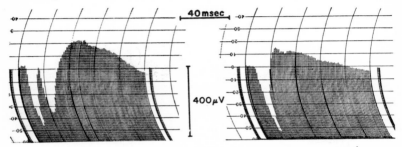

FIG. 78. RECORDS OF THE AVERAGE RESPONSE OF THE CAT'S
AUDITORY CORTEX TO A BRIEF CLICK

The envelope of each curve gives the average response of the auditory cortex to click stimuli sampled at 1 msec intervals. The preparation was an adult cat with a spinal transection at the level of the 1st vertebra. Clicks were delivered at the rate of 1/sec at an intensity 35 db above the threshold. Recordings were taken by means of a 'gross' concentric electrode with the outer electrode on the surface of the cortex and the inner electrode at a depth of 2 mm in the cortex. The left waveform shows the average cortical response without anaesthesia; the right waveform depicts the average response 1 hr after Dial (0·75 mg/Kg) had been injected intra-peritoneally. Computation was carried out by the electronic method of Barlow. The three pen deflections that stand alone at the beginning and end of each record are for calibration. The click was coincident with the first pen-stroke of the continuous curve.

(*By courtesy of Goldstein, Kiang and Brown.*)

the latter are transected in the cat at the level of the mid-brain, the animal can still be aroused from sleep by sounds.

These findings suggested to some that the function of the non-specific system might be the modification of central afferent transmission and that within its influence might lie the neuro-physiological mechanism responsible for 'listening' as contrasted with 'hearing'; this proposal recalls Adrian's suggestion of an 'editing' influence of the reticular formation on sensory inflow.

In fact some evidence that an electrophysiological difference can be detected between these two processes comes from the work of Galambos who finds potentials of increased amplitude in the auditory system of the cat when it is conditioned to expect a shock to follow the click. There are also the studies of Hernández Peón whose cats gave smaller responses (in the cochlear nucleus) to click when their attention was diverted from the sound by the presence of a live mouse. The interpretation of animal behaviour presents severe difficulties, and general enhancement of excitement may be a factor in experiments of this kind.

In some further work, Hernández Peón has shown that responses at the auditory cortex to monotonously repeated clicks die out after several thousand presentations and remain extinguished for many hours. He found that he could bring them back if he put the reticular formation out of action either reversibly by barbiturate anaesthesia or irreversibly by electro-coagulation.

This interpretation of a major controlling role for the reticular formation on the acoustically evoked response has been challenged from time to time. For example, the observed effect on responses of the cochlear nucleus to monotonously repeated stimuli is markedly reduced if the stimuli are presented through fixed earphones in order to eliminate the influence of sound-field variations in the environment of the test animal. An added complexity is the question, frequently raised, of the peripheral influence of the intrinsic ear muscles. That some reduction in the cochlear microphonic response results from reflex ear-muscle contraction has definitely been established, for these reflex contractions gradually relax during prolonged sound. Happily we are not deafened by our own vocalisations and this we owe, too, to our intrinsic ear-muscles, for they contract reflexly during the motor movements of articulation. In the light of these findings the task of sorting central from peripheral influences in such behavioural states as 'attention' and 'distraction' is clearly a formidable one.

Since the early anatomical observations of Held in the last century, it has been known that recurrent descending pathways exist in the auditory system, though only of late has their functional significance been appreciated. The schema proposed by Galambos and pictured on the right-hand side in

Fig. 77 depicts the supposed descending pathways. Later work has shown that although an efferent system lies in close proximity to the classic afferent pathway it is sufficiently separated from the latter to make it possible to stimulate at loci within it without activating the afferent neurones.

Evidence for central control by this descending efferent system with a strictly localised pathway has been presented by Desmedt. Stimulation at discrete loci in this system (mesial

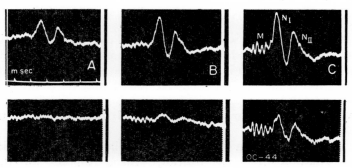

FIG. 79. INHIBITION OF AUDITORY NERVE RESPONSE BY HIGH-
FREQUENCY STIMULATION IN THE BRAIN STEM AT THE DECUSSATION
OF THE OLIVO-COCHLEAR BUNDLE

Upper 3 traces: Responses to clicks alone of intensity progressively increasing
from A to C. The nerve potentials are labelled N_1 and N_2 and the microphonic response M.
Lower 3 traces: Clicks delivered as in A, B and C but during high-frequency
stimulation of the olivo-cochlear bundle. Note suppression of neural
responses but not of the microphonic.
(From Galambos (1956) *J. Neurophysiol.*, **19,** 424.)

part of the ventral nucleus of the lateral lemniscus, ventral and anterior regions of the inferior colliculus and mesial portion of the medial geniculate) has been shown to suppress acoustically evoked potentials in the eighth nerve and in the cochlear nucleus. It was in the decussation of the olivo-cochlear bundle that Galambos had previously found an optimally effective locus for producing, by high-frequency stimulation, an inhibitory effect on responses of the auditory nerve to click. This effect is illustrated in Fig. 79.

The last link in the centrifugal path from the brain stem to the cochlea has been found anatomically by Rasmussen to pass in the olivo-cochlear bundle just beneath the 4th ventricle and then to run (alongside the afferent fibres of the 8th nerve) to the cochlea where its fibres are distributed to the whole length of the basilar membrane.

Whether these centrifugal fibres do in fact terminate on the hair cells themselves is not yet known, but they would certainly seem to be another form of central control over receptor response, analogous to the gamma efferent control over muscle spindles, outlined in Chapter 10. The demonstration of feedback control at the very points of contact of the organism with its environment is one of the major advances in sensory physiology in recent years, and one which calls for a further degree of sophistication in the stimulus-response concepts that have ruled for so long.

Earlier work in this field indicated that the topographically discrete response to different tones, initiated in the cochlea, were followed all the way through the brain where the pathways from the apex were found to connect, in the anaesthetised animal, with a different part of the auditory cortex than did those from the base responding to the high notes. In anaesthetised animals, Woolsey and Walzl mapped the areas of response in the cortex to electrical stimulation of the cochlear nerve in the cat, and Tunturi, using strychnine-evoked spikes, mapped them in the dog. In the cat, the response was found in the dorsal part of the anterior ectosylvian gyrus when stimulation was at the basal end of the cochlea, and in the posterior ectosylvian gyrus when stimulation was at the apex.

However, in unanaesthetised animals and with the modern techniques of unit recording, it has been demonstrated by several workers that neurones with widely differing characteristic frequencies are found together in quite small regions of the auditory cortex. The latter findings, which bring evidence against tonotopic representation in the cortex, would explain the behavioural studies that indicate that the auditory cortex of the cat is not concerned with frequency discrimination.

Each cochlea is represented in both hemispheres, and bilateral secondary projection areas with inverse pattern arrangements have also been located. This is in keeping with the secondary response areas found for the representation of other senses in the cortex, as noted in Chapter 1.

It should be remembered, however, that most of the classic

observations on localisation of response to acoustic stimuli were made on animals under anaesthesia. Modern knowledge tells us how misleading such 'maps' can be, and the development of techniques for recording from indwelling electrodes have revolutionised this field. As with other sensory systems, responses to stimuli of the receptor organ are evoked in association areas of the cortex outside what the anaesthetised animal led the early observers to regard as the sole receiving cortex.

At first sight it seems remarkable that the conducted nerve impulse, subscribing as it does to such well-defined limits of behaviour, should be able to convey so many aspects of sound, i.e. pitch, loudness, and the quality of timbre. Pitch, as has been seen, is conveyed essentially by the spatial characteristic of activity in the nerve pathways from its initiation in the sense organ to its destination in the auditory cortex. There is in addition a limited ability of the nerve fibre to respond to a given frequency of stimulus with a similar frequency of propagated impulses; this has in the single fibre a probable upper limit (imposed by the refractory period) of 500 impulses/sec, but, as has been mentioned, there is evidence that higher frequencies of the stimulus can be followed and it has been suggested that this might be effected by a rotational activation of fibres in the auditory nerve, individual fibres responding only to one in several sound-waves. It is, however, doubtful whether this property plays any role in the perception of pitch, since it is unlikely that such a 'following' would be carried faithfully through the synapses which lie between the auditory nerve and the cortex. It is an oversimplification to allot the sole cause of pitch discrimination to the place theory. Also, as has been noted, synchrony of discharge in different fibres may contribute to the sense of pitch for a given note, thus adding a time factor to the spatial one.

Intensity, as in other senses, is the essential characteristic conveyed by the frequency of impulses in the nerve fibre, the loudness of the stimulus correlating to some extent with the number of action spikes/sec.

From recordings of single units at various levels between the cochlea and the cortex, Katsuki has proposed that discrimination of frequency and intensity of sound (in the cat) may be made at the level of the medial geniculate body and that the function of the cortical area might be integration of the component sounds which had been analysed at the subcortical levels.

The discharge rate of most single units is certainly dependent on acoustic intensity, whether the unit be a neurone of the cochlear nerve or one in the cochlear nucleus, in the trapezoid body, the inferior colliculus, the medial geniculate nucleus or the auditory cortex, but subtle differences can be detected at each level in, for example: the degree of dependence of discharge rate and latency on stimulus frequency and stimulus intensity; the response cut-off at high frequencies; persistence of response to continuing sound; and degree of non-linearity of response to intensity.

Additionally, among auditory neurones, as in other systems in the brain, there are many units that emit a continuous discharge in the absence of external acoustic stimuli, and some of these respond to sound by a decrease in their activity. Some are unresponsive. Doubtless the patterning of excited, inhibited and silent neurones contributes a refinement of information transfer that a single, excitatory reaction could not convey.

At the cortex, if the sound stimulus is a continuous one, the characteristics of responses of single neurones tend to be (as in the visual system) either of the 'on' or 'off' or 'on-off' type, whereas at lower levels units usually continue to discharge for the duration of the stimulus. Clearly at the cortical level a new element has entered the coding system by which the brain receives information through its auditory system.

That the preceding statements may indeed be oversimplifications must always be borne in mind for, as in all single unit studies of the nervous system, the percentage of individual neurones from which direct recordings have been and are being made is so miniscule as to raise questions as to how meaningful their role is in 'the brain as a whole'. In order to understand the brain it is essential to learn the mechanisms of its components, but one must be chary in designing hypotheses on how the brain discriminates information from the behaviour of so few of its contributing neurones.

The qualities described as volume, timbre and density of sound fall in the realm of psychology. The compound form of the sound waves constituting any stimulus, is conveyed by the differential distribution of impulses of varied frequencies among the many fibres of the auditory nerve. The resultant

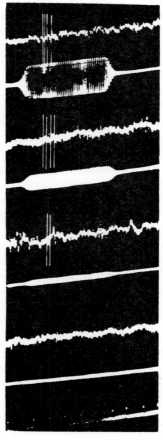

FIG. 80

On-type responses of a single cortical auditory neurone in an unanaesthetised and unrestrained cat to a tone burst of 7,000 c/s, in different intensities of 0, −10, −20 and −30 db respectively. Time in 0·01 sec is shown in lowest beam.

(From Katsuki (1960) *Electrical Activity of Single Cells.* Igaku Shoin.)

complex of different frequencies of discharge arriving in nerve paths originating in different levels of the basilar membrane gives the overall perception of a mixed sound. It is initially the variety of distribution and frequency of impulses in the 60,000 fibres of the two auditory nerves that is eventually elaborated into our perception of the many aspects of sound.

Theories of hearing have developed and changed as more and more facts have accumulated. Helmholtz's resonance theory of hearing, which explained the appreciation of pitch as a selective resonance due to differential tension at different levels of the basilar membrane, has been modified by other variations of the place theory. There is now, however, the definite evidence of Békésy that no such tension exists in the basilar membrane; a conclusion reached from direct observation of the membrane. The place theory retains the postulate that different portions of the basilar membrane vibrate selectively at different ranges of frequency but emphasises the role of progressive change in size of the anatomical structures from base to apex of the cochlea as decisive for this selectivity. The variation in width of the basilar membrane is the most important of these. The mass of the fluid in the cochlear canals also favours a topographical selection; a low frequency will set more fluid in motion than a high one, and a greater mass of fluid needs to be displaced to vibrate the basilar membrane at the apex than at the base of the cochlea.

A prevailing interest among electrophysiologists stems from the challenge to 'break the code' of information transfer in the central nervous system. High hopes have been placed by many in the auditory system for there, unlike the retina, the receptor is uncomplicated by chemical changes and has, as its first receptor neurone, a cell with an axon long enough to permit microelectrode recordings of its individual fibre-responses to varieties of acoustic stimuli. Considerable progress has been made in defining these peripheral responses to such qualities of the stimulus as frequency and intensity, but the transfer functions at each subsequent synapse still require elucidation.

Many workers have now obtained recordings which enable them to chart response curves for individual neurones at various stages of transfer through the brain. These usually depict, as an area on a graph of stimulus intensity versus frequency, all those frequencies that will produce a detectable response given sufficient intensity (see Fig. 81). The frequency at which a unit is most sensitive is the one requiring least

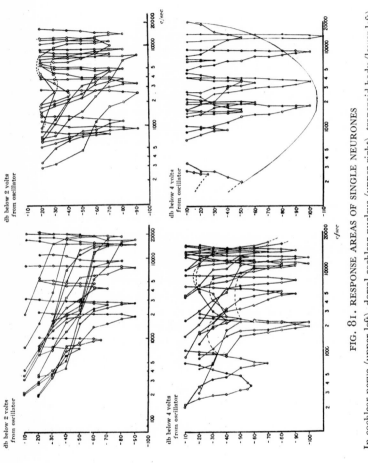

FIG. 81. RESPONSE AREAS OF SINGLE NEURONES

In cochlear nerve (upper left), dorsal cochlear nucleus (upper right), trapezoid body (lower left) and inferior colliculus (lower right). The curve without circles shows human threshold.

(From Katsuki and Uchiyama (1956) *Proc. imp. Acad. Japan*, **32**, 67.)

acoustic intensity to respond and is plotted as the low tip on the graph's contour; this is usually termed the 'characteristic frequency'.

Since the advent in the biological laboratory of computer analyses, much activity has gone into the analysis of the discharge patterns evoked in the units by stimuli of controlled parameters. Displays of these analyses have usually been in the form of bar graphs in which the frequency distribution of neuronal discharges is shown as a function of some variable. Essential as these studies are as a first step to understanding information transfer in the brain, much research lies ahead in designing less artificial experiments. Not only are the stimuli usually those rarely encountered in real life (clicks, tone bursts), but surgical exposure and electrode-tissue interface introduce yet other artefacts. The use of paralysing drugs or anaesthetics to immobilise the animal produces an imbalance of brain activity which must have its repercussions on the activity of its component neurones, as indeed does the impact of the anechoic environment in which most of these careful studies are made. These essential observations on isolated preparations need to be incorporated someday into the wider picture of information processing by the brain, but without them we cannot take the first step. As Kiang, one of the most active workers in this field, has said, 'It seems reasonable to adopt the position that psychophysiological judgements do not necessarily bear simple relationships to events at the level of the auditory nerve'.

BIBLIOGRAPHY

Barnes, W. T., Magoun, H. W. and Ranson, S. W. (1943) The ascending auditory pathway in the brain stem of the monkey. *J. comp. Neurol.*, **79**, 129–152.

Baust, W. and Berlucchi, G. (1964) Reflex response to clicks of cats' tensor tympanic during sleep and wakefulness and the influence thereon of the auditory cortex. *Arch. ital. Biol.*, **102**, 688–712.

Békésy, G. von (1960) *Experiments in Hearing*. McGraw-Hill, New York.

Békésy, G. von (1960) *Neural Mechanisms of the Auditory and Vestibular System*. Thomas, Springfield.

Békésy, G. von and Rosenblith, W. A. (1951) 'The Mechanical Properties of the Ear.' In *Handbook of Experimental Psychology*. Stevens (Ed.), Wiley, New York. Chapman and Hall, London.

Bremer, F. (1953) *Some Problems in Neurophysiology*. Athlone Press, London.

Buser, P. and Borenstein, P. (1959) Réponses somesthésiques, visuelles et auditives, recueillies au niveau du cortex 'associatif' suprasylvien chez le chat curarisé non anesthésié. *Electroenceph. clin. Neurophysiol.*, 11, 285–304.

Carmel, P. W. and Starr, A. (1963) Acoustic and non-acoustic factor modifying middle-ear muscle activity in waking cats. *J. Neurophysiol.*, 26, 598–616.

Davis, H. (1957) Biophysics and physiology of the inner ear. *Physiol. Rev.*, 37, 1–49.

Davis, H. (1959) 'Excitation of Auditory Receptors.' In *Handbook of Physiology—Neurophysiology*. Field, J., Magoun, H. W. and Hall, V. (Eds.) Vol. I. American Physiological Society, Washington.

Desmedt, J. E. (1960) 'Neurophysiological Mechanisms Controlling Acoustic Input.' In *Neural Mechanisms of the Auditory and Vestibular Systems*. Rasmussen, G. S. and Windle, W. F. (Eds.). Thomas, Springfield.

Desmedt, J. E. (1962) Auditory-evoked potentials from cochlea to cortex as influenced by activation of the efferent olivo-cochlear bundle. *J. acoust. Soc. Amer.*, 34, 1478–1496.

Evans, E. F., Ross, H. F. and Whitfield, I. C. (1965) The spatial distribution of unit characteristic frequency in the primary auditory cortex of the cat. *J. Physiol.*, 179, 238–247.

Fex, J. (1962) Auditory activity in centrifugal and centripetal cochlear fibers in cat. *Acta physiol. scand.*, 55, Suppl. 189.

French, J. D., Verzeano, M. and Magoun, H. W. (1953) An extra-lemniscal sensory system in the brain. *Arch. Neurol. Psychiat. (Chic.)*, 69, 505–518.

Galambos, R. (1944) Inhibition of activity in single auditory nerve fibres by acoustic stimulation. *J. Neurophysiol.*, 7, 287–303.

Galambos, R. (1954) Neural mechanisms of audition. *Physiol. Rev.*, 34, 497–528.

Galambos, R. (1956) Suppression of auditory nerve activity by stimulation of efferent fibres to cochlea. *J. Neurophysiol.*, 19, 424–437.

Held, H. (1893) Die centrale Gehörung. *Arch. Anat. Physiol. Anat. Abs.*, 201–248.

Helmholtz, H. von (1863) *Lehre von den Tonempfindungen*. Translated by Ellis, A. J. (1930) *Sensations of Tone*. Longmans, Green, New York.

Hernández Peón, R., Scherrer, H. and Jouvet, M. (1956) Modification of electrical activity in cochlear nucleus during 'attention' in unanesthetised cats. *Science*, **123**, 331–332.

Hind, J. E., Goldberg, J. M., Greenwood, D. D. and Rose, J. E. (1963) Some discharge characteristics of single neurons in the inferior colliculus of the cat. II. Timing of the discharges and observations on binaural stimulation. *J. Neurophysiol.*, **26**, 321–341.

Katsuki, Y. (1961) 'Neural Mechanism of Hearing in Cats and Insects.' In *Electrical Activity of Single Cells*. Y. Katsuki (Ed.). Igaku Shoin, Tokyo.

Kiang, N. Y-S. (1965) *Discharge Patterns of Single Fibres in the Cat's Auditory Nerve.* M.I.T. Press, Cambridge, Mass.

Lorente de Nó, R. (1933) Anatomy of the eighth nerve. *Laryngoscope* (St Louis), **43**, 1–38.

Nomoto, M., Suga, N. and Katsuki, Y. (1964) Discharge pattern and inhibition of primary auditory nerve fibres in the monkey. *J. Neurophysiol.*, **27**, 768–787.

Ramón y Cajal, S. (1911) *Histologie du système nerveux de l'homme et des vertébrés.* 2nd ed., 2 vols. Maloine, Paris.

Rasmussen, G. L. (1953) Further observations of the efferent cochlear bundle. *J. comp. Neurol.*, **99**, 61–74.

Rasmussen, G. L. and Windle, W. F. (Eds.) (1960) *Neural Mechanisms of the Auditory and Vestibular Systems.* Thomas, Springfield.

Rupert, A., Moushegian, G. and Galambos, R. (1963) Unit responses to sound from auditory nerve of the cat. *J. Neurophysiol.*, **26**, 449–465.

Snider, R. and Stowell, J. (1944) Receiving areas of the tactile, auditory and visual systems in the cerebellum. *J. Neurophysiol.*, **7**, 331–357.

Stotler, W. A. (1953) An experimental study of the cells and connections of the superior olivary complex of the cat. *J. comp. Neurol.*, **98**, 401–431.

Tasaki, I. (1954) Nerve impulses in individual auditory nerve fibres of guinea-pig. *J. Neurophysiol.*, **17**, 97–122.

Tunturi, A. R. (1944) Audio-frequency localisation in acoustic cortex of dog. *Amer. J. Physiol.*, **141**, 397–403.

Wever, E. G. (1949) *Theory of Hearing.* Wiley, New York.

Wever, E. G. and Bray, C. W. (1930) The nature of acoustic response: the relation between sound frequency and frequency of impulses in the auditory nerve. *J. exp. Psychol.*, **13**, 373–387.

Whitfield, I. C. (1957) The physiology of hearing. *Prog. Biophys.*, **8**, 1–48.

Woolsey, C. N. and Walzl, E. M. (1942) Topical projection of nerve fibres from local regions of the cochlea to the cerebral cortex of the cat. *Bull. Johns Hopk. Hosp.*, **11**, 315–344.

Worden, F. G., Marsh, J. T., Abraham, F. D. and Whittlesey, J. R. B. (1964) Variability of evoked auditory potentials and acoustic input control. *Electroenceph. clin. Neurophysiol.*, **17**, 524–530.

13

The Electrical Concomitants of
Smell and Taste

VERY little is known about the sense of smell compared with that of sight or hearing. The stimulus to the receptor cells is most generally regarded as the effect of inhaled particles dissolved in the moisture of the nose, although some work at Yale has led to the suggestion that the sense of smell may depend on radiation. According to this hypothesis the object being smelt absorbs certain wavelengths of the infra-red radiations from the sense organs in the nose and this change in radiation loss is thought to be interpreted by the brain as odour. Different receptor cells for different wavelengths are postulated to account for the appreciation of differences in smell. This concept of smell is not, however, generally accepted and at present lacks adequate evidence; moreover there is much that is incompatible, as, for example, the difference in smell between some (but not all) optical isomers. The more widely-accepted concept is that the olfactory cells are excited by direct contact with substances in solution.

When even the mode of stimulus can be so basically challenged, it is not surprising that little is known of the electrical activity associated with it. Smell is the only sensory system which does not have a primary projection to the thalamus (although there are some indirect interconnexions with the anterior thalamic nuclei). The nerve fibres in the 1st cranial nerve are unmyelinated and come directly from the sense cells in the mucous membrane of the olfactory cleft to the olfactory bulb. In the seventeenth century Thomas Willis had called these the 'smelling nerves' and noted that they were 'more remarkable in hunting Hounds than in any Animal whatsoever'. The fine structure of these C fibres received study by Gasser in the pig, using electron microscopy. In the olfactory

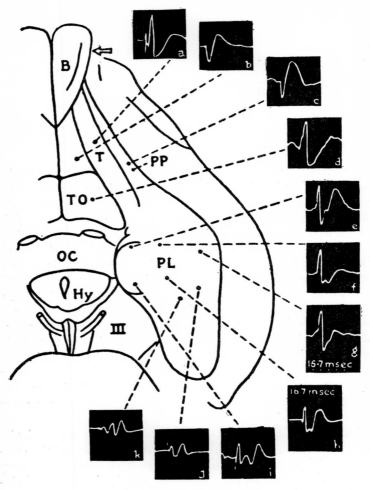

FIG. 82. BASAL VIEW OF THE CAT'S BRAIN SHOWING RESPONSES
EVOKED BY STIMULATION OF THE OLFACTORY BULB (AT THE OPEN
ARROW)

B, olfactory bulb; *PL*, pyriform lobe; *PP*, prepyriform cortex; *T*, lateral
olfactory tract; *TO*, olfactory tubercle.
Timeline in (*g*) applies to all records. Upward deflection indicates
negativity at the exploring lead.

(From Fox, McKinley and Magoun (1944) *J. Neurophysiol.*, **7**, 1.)

lobe several fibres from many olfactory cells impinge on the same secondary neurones. This concentration of many receptive messages on to few transferring pathways may explain the relative insensitiveness of this particular sense in man. For example with smell, a 30 per cent increase in intensity is necessary to produce a perceptible difference in sensation, whereas a 1 per cent change in a visible stimulus is detectable. In addition, the olfactory receptors occupy so small an area (only about 250 mm^2 bilaterally in man) in the upper part only of the nasal cavity that an ordinary inspiration usually fails to draw air past the sensory mucosa, and sniffing is necessary before they can be stimulated by anything but a very strong odour. The mitral and tufted cells in the olfactory bulb send their axons to the pyriform lobe, some fibres crossing in the anterior commissure to the olfactory bulb on the opposite side.

Electrophysiological studies of responses evoked by single shock stimulation of the olfactory bulb carried out by Fox, McKinley and Magoun located these in the prepyriform cortex, the anterior olfactory lobe, the olfactory tubercle and the pyriform lobe, but not in the hippocampus or septum (see Fig. 82). In fact the old theory that the latter structures were olfactory receiving areas is no longer tenable, for these electrophysiological findings have since received anatomical confirmation from Brodal.

At the receptor level, Ottoson recorded an electrical potential change in the olfactory mucosa of the frog when an odour-laden puff was blown into the nose. This consisted of a slow monophasic surface-negative potential, the rise-time and waveform of which were found to depend on the intensity of the odour. The slow potential rapidly adapts to continuous exposure to the same stimulus, though superimposed fast rhythmic waves may persist (Fig. 83). Similar long-lasting surface-negative responses of bullfrog olfactory epithelium to a jet of air saturated with butyl acetate have been found by Grundfest and others, who regard it as a generator potential in the receptors (although this interpretation has been challenged).

Adrian and others have demonstrated in animals the electrical response of the olfactory bulb to currents of air blown into the nose by inserting electrodes through the floor of the frontal sinus. In the absence of odours the bulb shows a continuous intrinsic activity consisting of waves of high frequency, usually about 100 per second. This rhythm is markedly affected by olfactory stimulation, though not by filtered air, thus mechanical stimulation of the receptors in the nasal mucosa apparently sends no messages to the olfactory bulb.

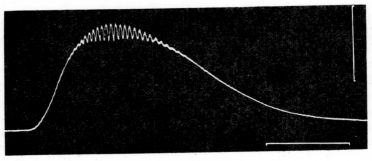

FIG. 83

Slow potential change with superimposed rhythmic waves recorded from the olfactory mucosa of the frog in response to amyl acetate. Vertical bar = 5 mV. Horizontal bar = 1 sec.
(From Ottoson (1956) *Acta. physiol. scand.*, Supplement, **35,** 1.)

Discharges in the bulb are greatly increased if the air inspired has been exposed to substances such as esters or hydrocarbons and oils, as has been demonstrated by Adrian in several species of animals (Fig. 84).

With concentrations of chemicals that give a just threshold stimulation, some neural basis has been found for qualitative differentiation of odours in the olfactory bulb as evidenced by the temporal and spatial distribution of potentials evoked in experimental animals. However, Adrian's studies of single fibre preparations suggest that this is only a preliminary sorting, inadequate to account for all the qualitative differentiations that can be made, and, on the quantitative side, Mozell's work in rabbits demonstrates that the spike discharges of the olfactory bulb are only crude indicators of intensity. It would seem that finer discriminations are made at a more central stage.

In man, recordings from the olfactory bulb have been made by Sem-Jacobsen and these studies have the added interest that subjective reports of the olfactory sensation could be obtained. The electrodes were too large to record activity of single units but the changes in frequency of the rhythmic potentials were felt to be compatible with some spatial distribution of zones responding maximally to certain odours.

As with other senses, the olfactory system has a supply of efferent fibres running centrifugally from the brain stem to the olfactory bulb. These fibres, which cross in the anterior commissure, have been known anatomically since the time of Ramón

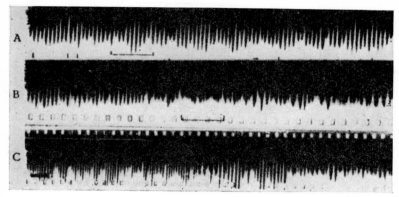

FIG. 84

Intrinsic waves at 100 c/s recorded from the olfactory bulb. *A:* in the absence of olfactory stimulus. *B:* weak stimulation by amyl acetate abolishes the rhythmic waves. *C:* strong stimulation with amyl acetate evokes a change in rhythm (rabbit).

(From Adrian (1950) *Electroenceph. clin. Neurophysiol.,* **2,** 337.)

y Cajal, but have only recently been explored electrophysiologically. Kerr and Hagbarth have found loci in the prepyriform cortex, the amygdala and the olfactory tubercle of the cat, that on stimulation by high frequencies depress the tonic discharge in the contralateral olfactory bulb as well as its response to odours. At low frequencies (e.g. 20/sec) there is contrastingly an enhancement of activity (Fig. 85). A similar effect can be obtained from stimulation of the anterior commissure in which these efferent fibres run. This is another example of centrifugal control over transmission of afferent impulses from a sense organ, analogous to those already described for the muscle spindle and the cochlea, and will be found described for the retina in Chapter 14.

Smell, like other senses, shows adaptation to a continuous stimulus, and an unchanging odour rapidly becomes unnoticed.

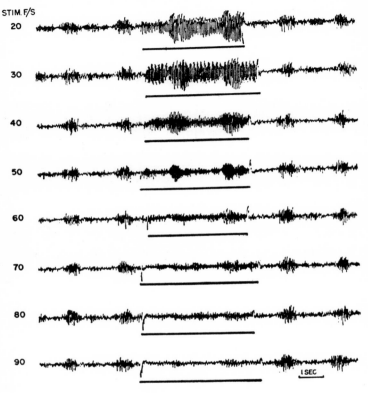

FIG. 85. CENTRIFUGAL CONTROL OF OLFACTORY IMPULSES.
RECORDINGS FROM OLFACTORY BULB OF A CAT RECEIVING
REPETITIVE OLFACTORY STIMULATION THROUGH A NASAL CATHETER

In those sections of the records that are underscored with black lines, the anterior commissure was stimulated electrically at a frequency shown on the left. At low frequencies there is an enhancement of discharge which undergoes transition as the frequency rises until at 90 c/s there is depression of activity.

(From Kerr and Hagbarth (1955) *J. Neurophysiol.*, **18**, 362.)

TASTE

Discussion of the sense of taste is hampered by the paucity of descriptive terms for it in the English language, but general agreement has been reached for the four clearly-marked tastes to which the human tongue is sensitive. These are described as salt, sour, bitter and sweet. It seems more likely that there is a differential response of the taste buds to combinations of these different stimuli than that there is a set of specific receptors exclusively sensitive to each.

The main stimulus for the taste described as 'salt' is the anion, as, for example, the Cl ion of a chloride or the SO_4 ion of a sulphate. The end-organs which respond maximally to salt are, in the human, the taste buds in the forward part of the tongue. The principal stimulus for 'sour' taste is the hydrogen ion of an acid and its effect is greatest at the side edges of the tongue. 'Sweet' substances, of which sugar is the obvious example, probably stimulate by reacting with lipoid substances in the taste buds and this possibly is also the mechanism for 'bitter' tastes, such as quinine. The human tongue is most sensitive to sweet tastes at the tip and to bitter at the back near the circumvallate papillæ.

The exact mechanism by which a chemical excites the sensory receptor is not known but, as with all other sense organs, the activity set up by the stimuli can be detected electrically in the afferent nerve. These studies are of necessity made on animals and an exact analogy to the human taste sense is not justifiable. For example, cats' tongues are apparently insensitive to sugar, a fact which no doubt explains why they prefer kippers to candy.

The taste buds, which consist of specialised primary neurones serving the highly-differentiated epithelial cells clustered in the papillæ of the tongue and more sparsely in the upper throat, are innervated by branches of three cranial nerves, the 7th, 9th and 10th. A branch of the 7th nerve, the chorda tympani, innervates the taste cells on the forward part of the tongue, the glosso-pharyngeal those at the back. A small area of taste buds in the region of the epiglottis is innervated by sensory fibres of the vagus.

Single fibre studies show that some serve sensory endings exclusively sensitive to acid ('sour'). Other single fibres show responses to both sour and salt, and yet a third type to both sour and bitter. It is possible that the single fibres in these latter cases innervate more than one type of taste receptor. In Fig. 86, the response, in the rat, of a single fibre specific to the chloride ion is seen to discharge increasingly rapidly as the concentration of NaCl was increased.

By gradually teasing out separate strands from the chorda tympani, Zotterman has demonstrated that each separate fibre has a specific pattern of sensitivity, though there are great differences among species as to the actual chemical substances that act as stimuli.

In Fig. 87 is one of Zotterman's records from a rhesus monkey. Several fibres are included in the strand, as can be

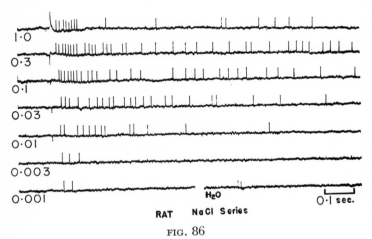

FIG. 86

Response of a single fibre of the chorda tympani nerve, sensitive to NaCl.
Note increase of discharge with increasing concentrations.
(From Pfaffman (1955) *J. Neurophysiol.*, **18**, 429.)

seen by the differing size of their discharges; this particular strand had been subdivided from a nerve that included also fibres from receptors sensitive to NaCl and to quinine.

The afferent pathway of the taste fibres is through cell stations in the solitary nucleus whose fibres cross to the opposite side and ascend in the medial lemniscus to the arcuate nucleus of the thalamus (nucleus ventralis posteromedialis). From this thalamic centre projection fibres for taste sensation go to the cortex near the lower end of the postcentral gyrus in the para-insular cortex of the opercular region. Thus, the pathways carrying taste sensation are found to travel very closely to those carrying somatic sensory impulses from the face. Changes in the electrical activity of this cortical area have been found by Ectors to follow chemical stimulation of the tongue in rabbits;

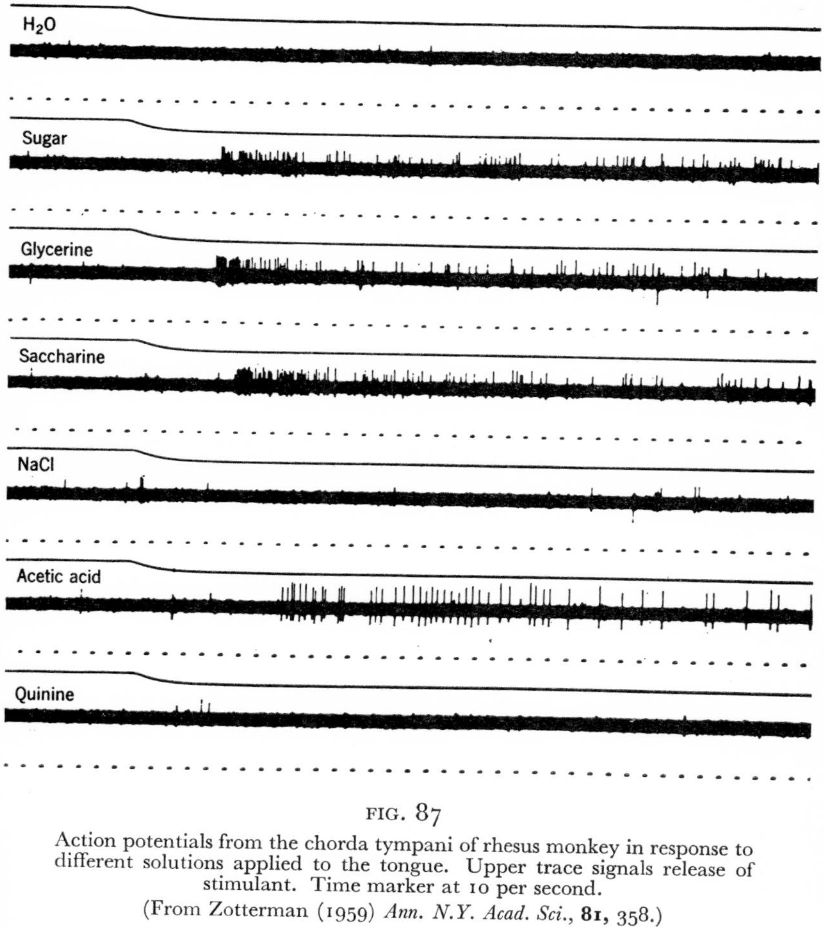

FIG. 87

Action potentials from the chorda tympani of rhesus monkey in response to different solutions applied to the tongue. Upper trace signals release of stimulant. Time marker at 10 per second.
(From Zotterman (1959) *Ann. N.Y. Acad. Sci.*, **81**, 358.)

conversely, electrical stimulation of this area has been found by Penfield to evoke a sensation of taste in man.

Chemical solutions are not the only stimuli to the tongue which set up action potentials in the afferent nerves: mechanical ones, such as brushing the tongue, produce impulses and so also do temperature changes. The action potentials of mechanical stroking and of chemical stimuli are, however, so different in amplitude that they cannot be confused; another distinguishing point is that impulses caused by the touch of a brush on the tongue cease when the brush is removed, whereas those from the chemical solution persist. The very great difference in amplitude suggests that the former impulses travel in the larger fibres from the touch receptors, while the action potentials from the taste cells are carried by the fine small fibres of the gustatory afferents which are only about 4μ in diameter. These two types of electrical response are seen very clearly in Fig. 88 from Pfaffman's work on the gustatory afferent impulses from the cat's tongue. A stronger chemical

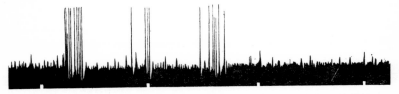

FIG. 88. THREE BURSTS OF LARGE POTENTIALS EVOKED BY BRUSHING THE TONGUE DURING A DISCHARGE OF SMALLER IMPULSES SET UP BY NaCl

Time signal: 0·25 sec.

(From Pfaffman (1941) *J. cell. comp. Physiol.*, **17**, 243.)

solution produces a greater frequency of discharge in the single nerve fibre up to a limiting maximal frequency.

Valuable information from human subjects has been obtained by Zotterman's group who have recorded from the chorda tympani in otosclerotic patients. The reported subjective estimates of the degree of sweetness corresponded closely with the magnitude of the summated response from the whole nerve. Similar correspondence between concentration and subjective estimate was also found for NaCl and for citric acid.

In general, the electrophysiological findings suggest that nuances of taste may be conveyed by the differential distribution of impulses of different frequencies in the several fibres of the gustatory nerve, the eventual sensation being a form of pattern recognition by the brain.

BIBLIOGRAPHY

Adey, W. R. (1959) 'The Sense of Smell.' In *Handbook of Physiology—Neurophysiology.* Field, J., Magoun, H. W. and Hall, V. (Eds) Vol. I. American Physiological Society, Washington.

Adrian, E. D. (1942) Olfactory reactions in the brain of the hedgehog. *J. Physiol. (Lond.),* **100,** 459–473.

Adrian, E. D. (1950) The electrical activity of the mammalian olfactory bulb. *Electroenceph. clin. Neurophysiol.,* **2,** 377–388.

Adrian, E. D. (1954) The basis of sensation: some recent studies of olfaction. *Brit. med. J.,* **i,** 287–290.

Allen, W. F. (1929) Effect on respiration, blood pressure and carotid pulse of various inhaled and insufflated vapours. *Amer. J. Physiol.,* **88,** 117–129.

Arduini, A. and Moruzzi, G. (1953) Sensory and thalamic synchronisation in the olfactory bulb. *Electroenceph. clin. Neurophysiol.,* **5,** 235–242.

Beck, L. H. and Miles, W. R. (1947) Some theoretical and experimental relationships between infra red absorption and olfaction. *Science,* **106,** 510.

Beidler, L. M. (1960) Physiology of olfaction and gustation. *Ann. Otol. (St Louis),* **69,** 398–409.

Benjamin, R. M. and Akert, K. (1959) Cortical and thalamic areas involved in taste discrimination in the albino rat. *J. comp. Neurol.,* **111,** 231–260.

Bornstein, W. S. (1940) Cortical representation of taste in man and monkey. *Yale J. Biol. Med.,* **12,** 719–736 and **13,** 133–156.

Brodal, A. (1947) The hippocampus and the sense of smell. *Brain,* **70,** 179–222.

Cohen, M. J., Landgren, L. S. and Zotterman, Y. (1957) Cortical reception of touch and taste in the cat. A study of single cells. *Acta physiol. scand.,* **40,** Suppl. 135.

Diamant, H., Oakley, B., Ström, L., Wells, C. and Zotterman, Y. (1965) A comparison of neural and psychophysical responses to taste stimuli in man. *Acta physiol. scand.,* **64,** 67–74.

Fox, C. A. McKinley, W. A. and Magoun, H. W. (1944) An oscillographic study of olfactory system of cats. *J. Neurophysiol.,* **7,** 1–16.

Gasser, H. S. (1956) Olfactory nerve fibres. *J. gen. Physiol.,* **39,** 473–496.

Gordon, G., Kitchell, R., Ström, L. and Zotterman, Y. (1959) The response pattern of taste fibres in the chorda tympani of the monkey. *Acta physiol. scand.,* **46,** 119–132.

Kerr, D. I. B. and Hagbarth, K-E. (1955) An investigation of olfactory centrifugal fibre system. *J. Neurophysiol.*, **18**, 362–374.

Moncrieff, R. W. (1944) *The Chemical Senses.* Leonard Hill, London.

Mozell, M. M. (1958) Electrophysiology of olfactory bulb. *J. Neurophysiol.*, **21**, 183–196.

Mozell, M. M. and Pfaffman, C. (1954) The afferent neural processes in odor perception. *Ann. N. Y. Acad. Sci.*, **58**, 98–108.

Ottoson, D. (1956) Analysis of the electrical activity of the olfactory epithelium. *Acta physiol. scand.*, **35**, Suppl. 122, 1–83.

Penfield, W. and Boldrey, E. (1937) Somatic motor and sensory representation in the cerebral cortex of man as studied by electrical stimulation. *Brain*, **60**, 389.

Pfaffman, C. (1941) Gustatory afferent impulses. *J. cell. comp. Physiol.*, **17**, 243–258.

Pfaffman, C., Erickson, R. P., Frommer, G. P. and Halpern, B. P. (1961) 'Gustatory Discharges in the Rat Medulla and Thalamus.' In *Sensory Communication.* Wiley, New York.

Sem-Jacobsen, C. W., Peterson, M. C., Dodge, H. W., Jacks, Q. D., Lazarte, J. A. and Holman, C. B. (1956) Electric activity of the olfactory bulb in man. *Amer. J. med. Sci.*, **232**, 243–152.

Sigg, E. B. and Grundfest, H. (1959) Pharmacological differences of similarly electrogenic neuraxial sites of bullfrog. *Amer. J. Physiol.*, **197**, 539–543.

Zotterman, Y. (1959) The nervous mechanism of taste. *Ann. N. Y. Acad. Sci.*, **81**, 358–366.

Zotterman, Y. (1961) 'Studies in the Neural Mechanism of Taste.' In *Sensory Communication.* Wiley, New York.

Zotterman, Y. (Ed.) (1963) *Olfaction and Taste.* Pergamon, Oxford; Macmillan, New York.

14

The Electrical Potentials of the
Visual System

THE primary receptor cells of the retina in man are morpho-
logically of two types: the cones, concentrated most densely
in the centre of the fovea, and the rods located outside this area.
The greater the distance from the fovea the smaller the ratio
of cones to rods, until in the extreme peripheral field scarcely
any cones are found. The names derive from the microscopic
appearance of the two types of cell and are more aptly descriptive of the shapes found in some animal eyes than in the human
eye. The cones are less responsive than rods to changes in
intensity of light, and in fact need considerable threshold
intensity before they will react at all, but they are extremely
sensitive to outline and to movement; they are also the
principal receptors for colour vision in man and in those
animals which are not colour-blind.

Although some differential sensitivity to wavelength has
been identified in the visual receptors of the cat, the rat and the
guinea-pig, there is no behavioural evidence for their having
colour vision that has gone unchallenged. There is, in fact,
no universally accepted evidence that the common laboratory
animals have colour vision nor, in spite of all the tales told by
the *aficionado*, has the bull. Primates are, in fact, the only
mammals other than man in whom colour vision has been
definitely proved, although it has been demonstrated beyond
reasonable doubt in several insects, fishes, and birds.

The rods react differently from the cones; they are very
sensitive to light, having a low threshold for intensity of illumination, and hence respond to a dim light or to any fluctuation
in the intensity of the light falling on the eye. This differentiation of two types of end-organ in the eye, each with a distinct
function, is the essence of the duplicity theory of vision as

originally formulated by Schultze and later by von Kries. More modern work, however, points to there being far more interplay between rod and cone mechanisms than the earlier workers supposed, and the allotment of cones to day vision and rods to night vision is now considered to be too simplified a concept of retinal function.

In man the visible part of the spectrum extends from about 4,000 Angström units (Å)* at the violet end to about 7,800 in the red (or even higher with very intense illumination). The peak of sensitivity for the cones in the light-adapted eye is in the yellow edge of the green band at about 5,600 Å. In the dark-adapted eye the maximal sensitivity of the rods is also in the green but the peak shifts to a blue-green at 5,000 Å. This effect, caused by a change from cone to rod vision, is called the Purkinje shift and was named for the eminent physiologist of Prague who, as a young man, described the phenomenon in his graduation thesis.

There is a different innervation for each of these two types of end-organ, as can be seen by the schematic drawing of Polyak's reproduced in Fig. 89, although again there is evidence for more interplay than is suggested by diagrams of this kind. Several rods are innervated by the same bipolar cell, hence many converge on to a single ganglion cell whose axon runs directly in the optic nerve. In the extreme peripheral field as many as 200 rods may make synaptic connexion with a single bipolar cell, which may therefore be triggered by quite slight changes in the intensity of the light striking the retina. The cones in the fovea have a more discrete innervation, hence can convey exactness of detail. In reptiles and birds, especially hawks which have great visual acuity, the fovea is very highly developed.

The action spikes of single ganglion cells in the retina have been recorded by microelectrodes, and some units have been differentiated that react to all the wavelengths of the visible spectrum in a way similar to that of the whole eye. Other units have been found that react only to certain bands of wavelengths. Granit has called the former type 'dominators' and the latter 'modulators'.

* An Angström unit, the standard measurement of wavelength, is one ten-millionth of a millimetre.

The mechanism by which the radiant energy of light changes the chemical composition of the receptor cell is not yet exactly known for cones, but has been worked out in some detail for

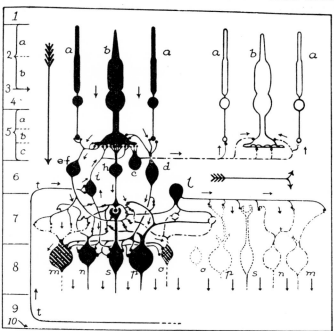

FIG. 89. POLYAK'S SCHEMATIC DIAGRAM OF THE RETINAL ELEMENTS AND SOME OF THEIR CONNEXIONS

a, rods; *b*, cones; *c*, horizontal cells; *d, e, f, h*, bipolar cells; *l*, amacrine cell; *m, n, s, p, o*, ganglion cells; *t*, centrifugal fibres. Arrows denote direction of conduction (see text).

The numbers on the left refer to the layers of the retina from 1, where the pigment epithelium lies, to 10 where the inner limiting membrane is found. The outer limiting membrane is at 3.

(From Polyak (1958) *The Vertebrate Visual System*. University of Chicago Press.)

rods. Rods in the vertebrate eye contain *rhodopsin*, a light-sensitive lipoprotein, commonly called visual purple, which was first described in the frog by Boll in 1876. The light-absorbing part of rhodopsin is vitamin A aldehyde which on exposure to light becomes bleached, but is restored during dark adaptation to its original form by enzymes in the retina. There is a direct relationship between the amount of unbleached visual purple in the rods and the sensitivity to light. This change in configuration of the vitamin A aldehyde is the only example where the molecular mechanism is known and is what apparently initiates the generator potential in the receptor cell.

A substance (called *iodopsin*) has been found in small quantities together with rhodopsin in the almost pure cone retina of chickens and is thought by Wald to be the light-sensitive element for the cones. The mechanism by which such chemical changes generate retinal action potentials is not known.

Because of the trichromatic nature of the human eye it has been postulated that at least three photosensitive pigments are likely to be present in the cones of the fovea. Of these Rushton has produced evidence for two.

The electrical concomitant of the response of the retina to light can be recorded as a mass response by registering the changes in the resting potential which always exists between the electronegative back of the eye and the electropositive cornea, so that current in an external circuit flows from the cornea to the fundus. This resting potential, which was discovered independently about a hundred years ago by Dewar and McKendrick in Edinburgh and by Holmgren in Uppsala, exists independently of illumination. In all eyes the free end of the visual cell is negative to its base and in the vertebrate eye, with which we are concerned here, the free end is at the fundus which is, therefore, negative to the cornea; in man, where the usual technique for recording electroretinograms is from an electrode on the cornea and another on the forehead, the corneal electrode is always positive to the forehead and becomes more so on illumination.

The electroretinogram was defined originally by Einthoven (and later by many workers) as the complex of potential variations contributed by at least three processes. These, as postulated by Granit, are shown in Fig. 90. The first effect to appear is the small negative *a*-wave. In this the cornea, which in the vertebrate eye is, as mentioned above, always positive to the fundus, becomes for a brief moment slightly less so. This initial decrease in the positivity of the cornea precedes a sudden marked increase (the positive *b*-potential) which is followed in the dark-adapted eye by a long slow surge of the same sign (the positive *c*-potential).

The resultant electroretinogram is the algebraic sum of these potential changes. Granit's analysis of the components of the electroretinogram was achieved largely through study of the differential effect of drugs. In fact, he named the components PI, PII, and PIII from the order in which these three components disappear with increasing depth of anaesthesia. Granit's second and third processes proved to be independent variables; for example, such drugs as atropine, eserine, and strychnine, all

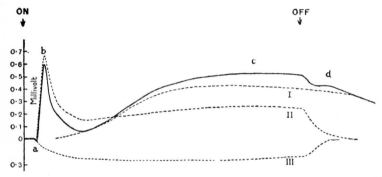

FIG. 90. THE ELECTRORETINOGRAM AND THE ANALYSIS OF ITS
COMPONENTS

(From Granit (1947) *Sensory Mechanisms of the Retina*. Oxford University
Press.)

of which affect the PII process, leave the PIII untouched. This is strong evidence that these components are contributed by different structures; he concluded that PII was an excitatory process and PIII an inhibitory one.

The origin of the first process, Granit's PI which is largely responsible for the prolonged *c*-potential, has not been determined, although it is known to be absent in the light-adapted eye. This process produces no discharge in the optic nerve and may be related in some way to the pigment epithelium. The second process, PII, is regarded by some as a reaction predominantly of the rods, though there is evidence that it is not exclusively so. This process produces the positive *b*-potential; in the dark-adapted eye part of this deflection is, as has been mentioned above, enhanced by the prolonged *c*-potential of the same sign. The third process, PIII, is, according to Granit, an inhibitory process which causes a negative deflection in the

electroretinogram at the beginning of illumination, the initial
a-potential. The opinion of some workers that this is exclusively
related to cone activity is not shared by Granit.

If the illumination has been both strong and prolonged, yet
another response is obtained when the light is shut off. This,
the *d*-potential, or 'off'-effect, takes the form of another positive
response followed by a slow return to the resting level as the eye
again becomes dark-adapted. This 'off'-effect, like the initial
'on' response to light (the *a*-potential), is much more prominent in the light-adapted than the dark-adapted eye, and is a
part of Granit's PIII process: a rebound on cessation of
illumination.

With increasing intensity of light the size of the *b*-wave
increases and its latency shortens (see Fig. 91). When a certain
intensity of illumination is reached, the *b*-wave ceases to gain
in amplitude though the *a*-wave becomes more marked. If the
area of retina illuminated is artificially restricted to less than
about 10 mm^2 (in the cat) a fully sized *b*-wave cannot be
elicited. Hence both intensity and area are important but
interchangeable factors.

In man, detailed studies of the electroretinogram have been
made by several workers including Monnier who has studied
the time relations of response in the retina and in the visual
cortex, a subject which is discussed more fully in Chapter 16
where the electrical activity of the brain is described.

A graded potential has been recorded in the retina by
Svaetichin who regards this as originating in the horizontal
cells and the Müller cells. As these are types of glial cells these
findings add to the current interest in the electrophysiology of
glia, much of which still remains controversial.

Electrical recording of impulses in single axons of an optic
nerve was first achieved by Hartline using the eye of the
horseshoe crab (*Limulus polyphemus*). In this invertebrate, the
fibres of the optic nerve are the axons of the receptor cells
themselves (the ommatidia) without the complexity of intermediate retinal neurones. In his single-unit analysis of the
nerve from this simple eye, Hartline was able to demonstrate
the logarithmic relation of frequency of the initial discharge to
intensity of illumination. The later finding, quoted by Granit,
that the potential difference across the ommatidium varies

logarithmically with intensity of illumination and directly with impulse frequency makes it highly likely that this is the mechanism for generating propagated impulses in the optic nerve of these animals. Even in this comparatively simple eye, however,

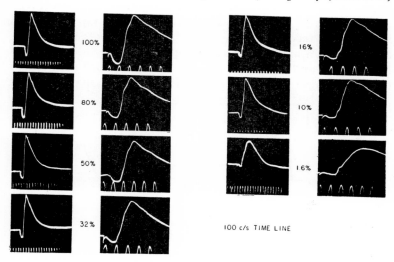

FIG. 91. THE EFFECT OF CHANGING INTENSITY ON THE
ELECTRORETINOGRAM OF THE CAT

The intensity was lowered by the use of filters each of which introduced a measured percentage reduction in illumination. The unfiltered source of white light was therefore given the arbitrary designation of 100 per cent and the subsequent reductions in illumination are entered as percentages opposite the electroretinograms to which they refer. The flash was 32 μsec in duration.

Two sweep speeds are shown for each degree of illumination: on the right a fast sweep to indicate latencies. Time line in all records: 100 c/s. Amplification constant for all records. At even fainter illumination than that used here there may be no trace of an *a*-wave.

(From Brazier (1954) *Electroenceph. clin. Neurophysiol.*, Supplement, **4**, 93.)

the action of a receptor cell is not independent of its neighbours, activity of which may exert an inhibitory influence. This interplay is not in the receptor cells themselves but is an interaction between their nerve fibres in the plexus just behind the ommatidia.

Of great interest is the question of how the visual stimulus is coded as a pulse pattern in the optic nerve. A great deal is now known in the case of the *Limulus* eye, where a single nerve fibre serves a single photoreceptor but, unfortunately, the vertebrate eye is far more complex as a glance at Fig. 89 will reveal.

In the discussion above of the electroretinogram, note was made of the off-response. In 1927 Adrian and Matthews (working with the eel) showed that an off-response could similarly be recorded from the (whole) optic nerve (Fig. 92), and since then single fibres and receptors serving these responses have been found in several species. The first to be found was in the frog where Hartline dissected out fibres carrying three

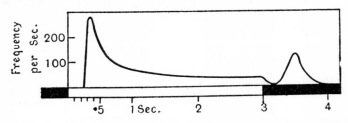

FIG. 92. FREQUENCY OF IMPULSES PER SEC DURING AND AFTER STEADY ILLUMINATION OF THE EYE OF AN EEL

The duration of lighting is shown by the white band below the baseline.
(From Adrian and Matthews (1927) *J. Physiol. (Lond.)*, **63**, 378.)

common classes of response in the optic nerve: those that discharge at the onset of illumination and continue throughout it, others that discharge only at its cessation, and yet others that respond briefly to both 'on' and 'off'. Fibres showing adaptation to continuing illumination were commonly found (see Fig. 93). Further analysis revealed the inhibiting effect on an off-response of re-illumination. The development of techniques by which recordings can be made from micro-electrodes in the ganglion cells in the retina (see Fig. 94) has confirmed the findings first made in their axons (namely the three broad categories of response) and has provided the added information that units may change their category with varying intensity and wavelength (at least in the cat). It should therefore be the balance of activity in the receptor field that is categorised rather than the fibres that bear the resultant message. In this way a greater plasticity is available than could be achieved by rigid ganglion or fibre types.

Opportunity for a greater subtlety of interaction in the retina than the above findings would suggest is provided by the fact that the receptor field of a single ganglion cell overlaps those of others (as indeed the histology would demand). By using a very small light spot as his stimulus, Kuffler demonstrated in the cat that the area of retina that has to be illuminated in order for a single ganglion cell to discharge, has more or less concentric zones where each of the three categories of response are represented, some with a central zone for 'on', some with a

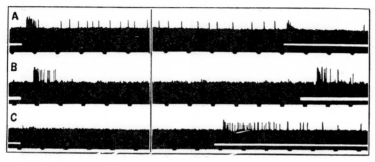

FIG. 93. THREE TYPES OF IMPULSE DISCHARGE FROM SINGLE FIBRES OF THE OPTIC NERVE OF THE FROG

A, maintained response; *B*, on-and-off response; *C*, off response. The occlusion of the white horizontal bar in each record indicates the period of illumination. Time signal: 1–5 sec.

(From Hartline (1938) *Amer. J. Physiol.*, **121**, 400.)

central zone for 'off'. In either case the fringe of the receptor field is usually inhibitory to the activity of its centre (Fig. 95). Microelectrode recordings from various sense organs have revealed that they have a maintained activity in the absence of observable external stimulation, and the retina is no exception. It is conceivable therefore that an additional mechanism through which the brain can receive information is by departure of the message from a predictable discharge, 'meaning' being introduced by the degree of probability exceeding chance.

Among the phenomena that were first observed in recordings from lower animals in response to retinal illumination was an oscillatory response in the optic nerve. More recent studies with recordings from microelectrodes in single fibres of the optic tract have shown these oscillatory potentials to be synchronous with grouped discharges in individual axons, and suggest an alternating facilitation and inhibition in the parent ganglion cells located in the retina.

In the mammalian optic nerve (cat or rabbit) when the response to electrical stimulation is recorded from the whole

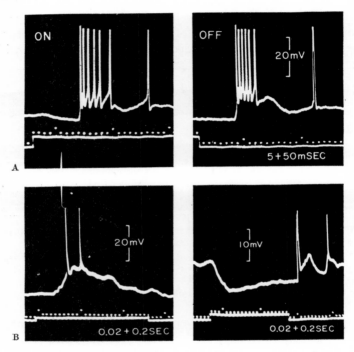

FIG. 94. RECORDINGS FROM SINGLE NEURONES IN THE FROG'S RETINA

The two upper photographs (*A*) are from the same neurone showing its response both to 'on' and 'off' of the light. *B* is from a neurone that responded to 'on' only, and *C* to 'off' only.

(From Tomita, Marakani, Hashimoto and Sasaki (1961) In *Visual System: Neurophysiology and Psychophysics.* Springer.)

nerve the action potential is found to be predominantly bimodal, for there are at least two main groupings of fibre sizes conducting at different rates (Fig. 96). When a flash is used as the stimulus, recordings of the compound action potential of the optic nerve behind the eyeball usually include some electrotonic spread into the nerve of the electroretinal potential.

Since this is cornea-positive its invasion of the nerve appears as a slow positive deflection larger in size the closer the electrodes are to the eye.

Not all the fibres of the optic tract synapse in the lateral geniculate, for some pass through the medial border and continue to the brain stem to serve the pupillary reflex (Fig. 97). The fibres mediating this reflex were shown by Magoun and

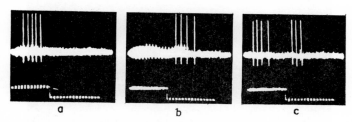

a   b   c

FIG. 95. SINGLE-UNIT RECORDINGS FROM GANGLION CELLS IN THE CAT'S RETINA

A light spot 0·2 mm in diameter evoked an 'on' response in ganglion cell at region *a*. At position *b*, 0·5 mm away, the same stimulus evoked 'off' responses. In the region *c*, between *a* and *b*, an 'on-off' response was obtained.

Lower beam signals intensity and duration of light flash. Time base given by 50/sec breaks in signal line. Amplitude of unit discharges: 0·5 mV.

(From Kuffler (1953) *J. Neurophysiol.*, **16**, 37.)

Ranson to terminate in the pretectal region of the brain stem and not, as originally thought, in the superior colliculus. Second order neurones make the connexion with cells of the 3rd nerve nucleus which are responsible for the efferent limb of the pupillary reflex arc. Electrical responses can be obtained in the pretectal region with lower thresholds of stimulation than are required for the superior colliculus, and are hence presumably carried by larger fibres. The superior colliculus is in fact activated by retinal illumination through multiple routes, including contributions from the optic nerve, and transsynaptically from other regions of the brain stem and from the cortex, and has been shown to be involved in eye-movements (as are other brain stem sites). The electrical sign of the responses of the colliculus to a brief flash is a slow wave-like discharge suggestive of a polyneuronal pathway, and its

latency is longer (by several msec) than that of the response at
the cortex.

The thalamic relay station for the visual system, the lateral
geniculate nucleus, is a laminated structure and the connexions

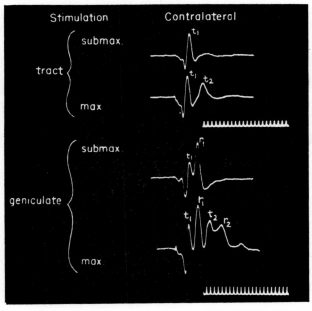

FIG. 96

Recordings from optic tract and lateral geniculate nucleus of cat during
electrical stimulation of the optic nerve. At submaximal current strength
only the low threshold fibres respond (t_1). Their response is also recorded
at their entry into the geniculate (t_1) together with the postsynaptic
response of the geniculate neurones (r_1). At maximal stimulation strength
the higher threshold fibres of the tract also respond (t_2) and evoke a second
postsynaptic response (r_2). Time marker: 0·2 msec.

(From Bishop and McLeod (1954) *J. Neurophysiol.*, **17**, 391.)

that have been found histologically can be demonstrated
electrophysiologically. For example, in the three-layered
geniculate of the cat the outer two layers give responses to
illumination of the contralateral eye, the middle layer to
illumination of the ipsilateral eye.

The earlier concept of the lateral geniculate nucleus being
merely a way-station that relayed its input from the optic

nerve transynaptically to the cortex is no longer tenable, for
this is not its sole input. There are neurones in the reticular
formation that terminate in the lateral geniculate and it is
doubtless these that carry the impulses that modify the activity
of these thalamic neurones during states of arousal, and account

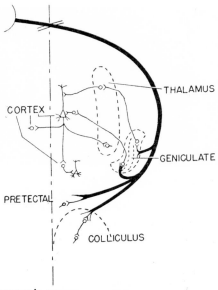

FIG. 97. BISHOP'S SCHEMATIC DIAGRAM OF FOUR SUGGESTED
PATHWAYS FROM THE CONTRALATERAL EYE OF A CAT

They are (a) lateral geniculate → radiations → Golgi type II neuron →
axo-somatic synapsis with pyramidal cell cortex. (b) geniculate → non-
specific thalamic relay → axo-dendritic synapsis with apical dendrite of
cortical cell. (c) pretectal region. (d) superior colliculus.

(From original of Fig. 6, Bishop and Clare (1955) *J. comp. Neurol.*, **103,** 295.)

for the changes in the amplitude of visually evoked responses in
conditions of 'attention' and 'distraction'.

By the time visual impulses reach the cortex their electrical
sign has become more complex. The most detailed analyses
have been made in the cat, where the response to a single
volley to the optic nerve, geniculate or radiations, is a series of
four surface-positive spikes, all but the first of which ride on a
slow diphasic (positive-negative) wave (see Fig. 98). Bishop has
identified the first spike as the action potentials of the axons of

the geniculate cells and the subsequent ones as postsynaptic responses of neurones within the cortex activated serially.

The response of the visual cortex to flash can be recorded in man, though the presence of the skull and the inaccessibility of the calcarine cortex often makes these potentials difficult to

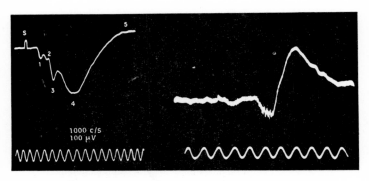

FIG. 98. THE RESPONSE AT THE VISUAL CORTEX OF THE ANAESTHETISED CAT TO STIMULATION OF THE OPTIC NERVE; MACROELECTRODE RECORDINGS

Left: Response to a volley. The numbers relate to Bishop's analysis of the sequence of events according to which: 1 = radiation spike; 2 = Golgi II discharge; 3 = discharge of pyramidal cells in deep layers of the cortex initiating the slow diphasic wave of the basal dendrites, initially surface-positive becoming surface-negative by electronic invasion of the apical dendrites; 4 = spike discharge of pyramidal cells in more superficial cortical layers (largely masked in this recording by the dendritic wave). Surface negativity upwards.

(From Malis and Kruger (1956) *J. Neurophysiol.*, **19**, 172.)

Right: Response to a brief flash. The diffusing action of the retina scatters the initial spikes but the slow diphasic wave can still be recorded at the cortex. Time line: 200 c/s. Light pentobarbital anaesthesia. Flash indicated by small notch.

(From Brazier (1954) *Conference on Neuropharmacology.* Vol 1, 107. Josiah Macy Jr. Foundation, New York.)

detect among the background activity of the electroencephalogram. Techniques are, however, now available for averaging a series of responses and these delineate the potential changes with considerable clarity (Fig. 99). As Bishop and O'Leary showed a long time ago in the rabbit, the initial response may be followed by an after-discharge resembling a train of alpha waves. The same phenomenon is found in man, and averaging techniques that preserve information about phase relationship between the flash and the peaks of these waves show them to be phase-locked to the stimulus.

When looked at with a faster time course many details emerge in the earlier part of the trace, especially if a number of responses are averaged by a computer in order to de-emphasise the on-going electroencephalographic potentials

(AVERAGE OF 180 RESPONSES)

0   85   170 225 milliseconds

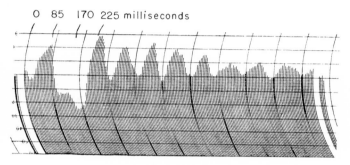

FIG. 99. RESPONSE TO FLASH IN MAN

The envelope of the curve gives the average of 180 responses at 5-msec intervals and recorded by unipolar linkage from the occipital region of the skull. The first three pen deflections that stand alone on the left, and the detached group on the right are for calibration of the base line. The flash was coincident with the first pen deflection of the continuous series. Note early occipital-positive response followed by large negative-positive complex and the rhythmic after-discharge phase-locked to the flash. Electronic averager designed by Barlow.

(From Brazier (1958) *Symposium on Electroencephalography and Higher Nervous Activity*. Academy of Sciences, U.S.S.R.)

that may mask the evoked response in man. The earliest potential change evoked in the light is usually between 25 and 35 msec, as first demonstrated by Cobb; this is then followed by many other components. There are many indi-vidual differences in these details and, of course, the waveform will depend on the placement on the scalp from which the recording is made. In Fig. 100, the average response to 300 flashes in an unanaesthetised man as recorded from a central-occipital linkage is shown.

The major part of the early pioneer work on the electro-physiological characteristics of the visual pathway have been tests of responses in animals (with fixed pupils) to the sudden onset of a bright light, an event that we experience almost only when facing the photographer's flash-bulb. In addition, the mammalian eye does not have a fixed gaze and these incessant uncontrollable eye movements must influence receptive fields in the retina. Modern research has therefore turned to the use of stimuli such as moving spot or contour and this has yielded results of very great interest. Neurones in the cat's visual cortex, unresponsive to a light flash, have been shown to be

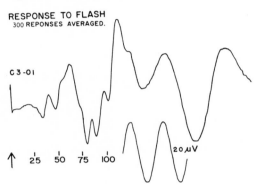

FIG. 100. AVERAGE WAVEFORM OF 300 RESPONSES TO FLASH
RECORDED FROM A NORMAL MAN

The various components of the waveform have different fields on the surface of the scalp and therefore give their maximum amplitude at different sites on the head.

activated by flicker, others by moving stimuli and yet others by patterned light at the contrasting edges between light and dark.

Experiments of this type have been intensely pursued by the Freiburg School who originally proposed a classification into 5 types of neuronal response in the visual cortex of the cat, as depicted schematically in Fig. 101. The exact borders in this classification into 5 types of unit response become less clear in the unanaesthetised animal in whom reticulo-thalamic influences are unimpaired and activity in collateral fibres preserved. However, these basic differentiations have proved useful as the basis for greater refinements and have been applied to other stations in the visual pathway.

The behaviour of any individual unit being recorded is always under the influence of its neighbours: i.e. by reciprocal inhibition of neurones in the same region and lateral inhibition of synergistic neurones in surrounding regions. Lateral inhibition in receptive fields is a well-established phenomenon

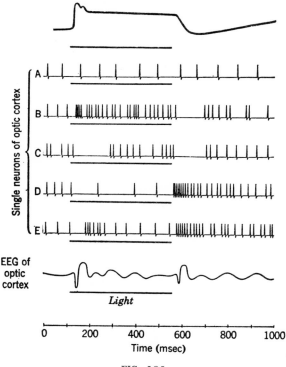

FIG. 101

Schematic display of five types of neuronal response found in the cat's visual cortex. *A*: Unresponsive. *B*: Activated by light, inhibited by dark (on-response). *C*: Inhibited by both light and dark. *D*: Activated by dark (off-response). *E*: Delayed activation by light, immediate activation by dark (on-off response).

(From Jung, Creutzfeldt and Grüsser (1958) *Germ. med. Mth.*, **3**, 269.)

in the retina and can be demonstrated in other stations of the visual pathway. In the case of the retina some specialised receptive fields may also be detected (in the cat).

Clear evidence for surround inhibition in the cat's lateral geniculate nucleus has been demonstrated by Hubel, as illustrated in Fig. 102. This shows a unit which responded with a marked high frequency discharge when a small locus in the visual field was brightly lighted but ceased to fire when the spot itself was darkened and the surrounding area illuminated.

Reversal of response in changing from a bright to a dark field has been demonstrated at early stages in the visual pathway as, for example, by the work of Kuffler and his associates in the retina. That there may be directional differentiation by individual neurones is supported by the findings of Barlow and Hill in the retina of the rabbit, where movement of the

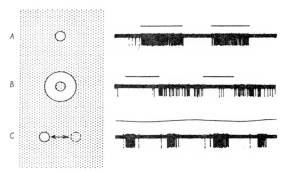

FIG. 102

Intracellular recordings from a unit in the cat's lateral geniculate nucleus. When a point of light was moved across the retina this unit responded only when the light was positioned as shown in *A*. If, instead, the same spot was darkened and a ring surrounding it lighted (as in *B*) the unit ceased to fire during illumination and gave only 'off' responses. The effect of moving the light spot horizontally backwards and forwards across the receptive field of this neurone is shown in *C*. The line above each record indicates when the light was on.

(From Hubel (1960) *J. Physiol.* (*Lond.*), **150**, 91.)

object in one direction activates a discharge but reversal of direction evokes no response.

In the lateral geniculate nucleus the contrasting reaction of neurones is also very striking, as has been brought out by the work of Baumgartner. Neurones have been demonstrated which are maximally activated by a black-white contrast, the number of discharges being markedly greater than those evoked by an all-white field.

Similar differences of behaviour among the neurones of the cat's visual cortex are brought out by a patterned stimulus of bright-dark stripes. The reaction of those neurones essentially activated by brightness is in strong contrast to those that react to darkness (the so-called B and D neurones according to the nomenclature of the Freiburg school).

Even more striking, in terms of the animal's natural experiences outside the laboratory, are the recent data on movement perception. The reactivity of neurones in the cat's visual

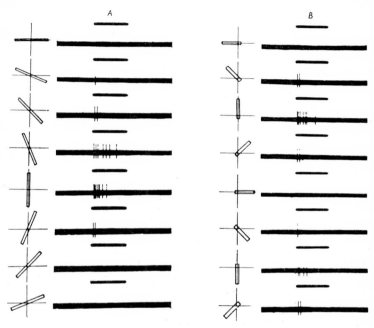

FIG. 103

Responses of a single neurone in the cat's visual cortex to changing orientation of a rectangular slit of light. Note that on rotation of the slit the unit was maximally activated when the slit reached the vertical orientation and was inhibited by horizontal position. Angular orientations have intermediate discharge counts.

(From Hubel and Wiesel (1959) *J. Physiol. (Lond.)*, **148,** 574.)

cortex to moving bright-dark bars has revealed differentiating responsivity to the orientation of these edge effects. In an extensive research on this problem Hubel and Wiesel have been able to define complex units which respond to a particular orientation of the stimulus irrespective of where it is placed in the visual field (Fig. 103).

Exploration of intracellular responses of individual neurones in the cat's visual cortex on stimulation of the lateral geniculate body have led Li to the conclusion that inhibitory as well as excitatory fibres project from this nucleus on to cortical cells, for units were found which responded only with hyperpolarisation, others with depolarisation alone.

Clear demonstrations have been made of the convergence on to the same cortical neurone by both retinal illumination and stimulation of the non-specific thalamus though, not unexpectedly, the latencies of response differ. It has been proposed that the impulses reaching the cortical neurone via the lateral geniculate make axo-somatic connexions, whereas the non-specific afferents make contact through axo-dendritic synapses and play a role as modulators.

In previous chapters some mention has been made of centrifugal control over sense receptors as evidence by activity in the gamma efferent fibres to muscle spindles and in the olivocochlear bundle, and by central influence over discharges in the olfactory bulb. Another example is found in the retina where Granit has demonstrated a change in rate of retinal cell discharge following stimulation of the reticular substance of the brain stem. Both inhibitory and facilitatory influences on single retinal neurones have also been elicited by Granit by stimulation at other stations in the brain stem (for example, in the superior colliculus and from fibre tracts just above it).

It is difficult to explain such a result on any basis except a return pathway including neurones within the brain stem, although the anatomical identification of their cell bodies has not yet been made. Efferent fibres entering the retina have, however, been known since Ramón y Cajal's demonstration of them in the dog.

The demonstration of this type of control exerted at the receptor is one of the newer developments in the physiology of the sense organs and one that brings with it need for a reconsideration of mechanisms underlying the integration of the nervous system.

BIBLIOGRAPHY

Adrian, E. D. and Matthews, R. (1927) The action of light on the eye. The discharge of impulses in the optic nerve and its relation to electric changes in the retina. Part I. *J. Physiol. (Lond.)*, **63**, 378–414.

Ajmone Marsan, C. and Morillo, A. (1963) Callosal and specific response in the visual cortex of cat. *Arch. ital. Biol.*, **101**, 1–29.

Barlow, H. B., Fitzhugh, R. and Kuffler, S. W. (1957) Change or organisation in the receptive fields of the cat's retina during dark adaptation. *J. Physiol. (Lond.)*, **137**, 338–354.

Barlow, H. B. and Hill, R. M. (1963) Selective sensitivity to direction of movement in ganglion cells of the rabbit retina. *Science*, **139**, 412–414.

Bartley, S. H. (1941) *Vision*. Van Nostrand, New York; Macmillan, London.

Baumgartner, G. and Hakas, P. (1962) Die Neurophysiologie des simultanen Helligkeitskontrastes. *Pflügers Arch. ges. Physiol.*, **274**, 489–510.

Bishop, G. H. and Clare, M. H. (1951) Radiation path from geniculate to optic cortex in cat. *J. Neurophysiol.*, **14**, 497–505.

Bishop, G. H. and Clare, M. H. (1953) Sequence of events in optic cortex response to volleys of impulses in the radiation. *J. Neurophysiol.*, **16**, 490–498.

Bishop, P. O., Burke, W. and Davis, R. (1962) The identification of single units in central visual pathways. *J. Physiol. (Lond.)*, **162**, 409–431.

Bremer, F. (1956) Analogie remarquable des réponses sensorielle et collosale de l'aire visuelle du chat. *Arch. int. Physiol. Biochim.*, **64**, 234–250.

Bremer, F. and Stoupel, N. (1959) Facilitation et inhibition des potentiels évoqués corticaux dans l'éveil cérébral. *Arch. int. Physiol. Biochim.*, **67**, 240–275.

Brindley, G. S. (1960) *Physiology of the Retina and the Visual Pathway*. Arnold, London.

Brindley, G. S. and Gardner-Medwin, A. R. (1966) The origin of the early receptor potential of the retina. *J. Physiol. (Lond.)*, **182**, 185–194.

Brown, P. K. and Wald, G. (1964) Visual pigments in single rods and cones of the human retina. *Science*, **144**, 45–52.

Cigánek, L. (1961) The EEG response (evoked potential) to light stimulus in man. *Electroenceph. clin. Neurophysiol.*, **13**, 165–172.

Cobb, W. A. and Morton, H. B. (1952) The human retinogram in response to high-intensity flashes. *Electroenceph. clin. Neurophysiol.*, **4**, 547–556.

Cobb, W. A. and Dawson, G. D. (1960) The latency and form in man of the occipital potentials evoked by bright flashes. *J. Physiol. (Lond.)*, **152**, 108–121.

Cole, J. (1953) The relative importance of colour and form in discrimination learning of monkeys. *J. comp. Psychol.*, **15**, 16–18.

Dewar, J. and McKendrick, J. G. (1873) On the physiological action of light. *Trans. roy. Soc. Edinb.*, **27**, 141–166.

Dodt, E. and Wirth, A. (1953) Differentiation between rods and cones by flicker electroretinography in pigeon and guinea pig. *Acta physiol. scand.*, **30**, 80–89.

Doty, R. W. and Kimura, D. S. (1963) Oscillatory potentials in the visual system of cats and monkeys. *J. Physiol. (Lond.)*, **168**, 205–218.

Dowling, J. E. (1963) Neural and photochemical mechanisms of visual adaptation in the rat. *J. gen. Physiol.*, **46**, 1287–1301.

Dumont, S. and Dell, P. (1958) Facilitations spécifiques et non-spécifiques des réponses visuelles corticales. *J. Physiol. (Paris)*, **50**, 261–264.

Fuortes, M. G. F. (1959) Initiation of impulses in visual cells of limulus. *J. Physiol. (Lond.)*, **148**, 14–28.

Fuortes, M. G. F. and Yeandle, S. (1964) Probability of occurrence of discrete potential waves in the eye of limulus. *J. gen. Physiol.*, **47**, 443–461.

Fuortes, M. G. F. and Hodgkin, A. L. (1964) Changes in time scale and sensitivity in limulus ommatidia. *Docum. ophthal. (Den Haag)*, **18**, 284–286.

Granit, R. (1947) *Sensory Mechanisms of the Retina*. Oxford University Press, London.

Granit, R. (1955) *Receptors and Sensory Perception*. Yale University Press, New Haven.

Grüsser, V., Grüsser, O-J. and Bullock, T. H. (1963) Unit responses in the frog's tectum to moving and non-moving visual stimuli. *Science*, **141**, 820–822.

Hartline, H. K. (1938) The response of single optic nerve fibers of the vertebrate eye to illumination of the retina. *Amer. J. Physiol.*, **21**, 400–415.

Hartline, H. K. and Ratliff, F. (1956) Inhibitory interaction of receptor units in the eye of limulus. *J. gen. Physiol.*, **40**, 357–376.

Hernández-Peón, R., Guzmán Flores, C., Alcaraz, M. and Fernández Guardiola, A. (1957) Sensory transmission in visual pathway during 'attention' in unanesthetised cats. *Acta neurol. Lat.-amer.*, **3**, 1–8.

Holmgren, F. (1865–6) Über die Retinaströme. *Upsala Läk.-Fören. Förh.*, **1**, 177–181.

Hubel, D. H. (1958) Cortical unit responses to visual stimuli in nonanesthetised cats. *Amer. J. Ophthalmol.*, **46**, 110–122.

Hubel, D. H. (1959) Single unit activity in striate cortex of unrestrained cats. *J. Physiol. (Lond.)*, **147**, 226–238.

Hubel, D. H. (1960) Single unit activity in lateral geniculate body and optic tract of unrestrained cats. *J. Physiol. (Lond.)*, **150**, 91–104.

Hubel, D. H. and Wiesel, T. N. (1959) Receptive fields of single neurones in the cat's striate cortex. *J. Physiol. (Lond.)*, **148**, 574–591.

Hubel, D. H. and Wiesel, T. N. (1962) Receptive fields, binocular interaction and functional architecture in the cat's visual cortex. *J. Physiol. (Lond.)*, **160**, 106–154.

Hubel, D. H. and Wiesel, T. N. (1963) Shape and arrangement of columns in cat's striate cortex. *J. Physiol. (Lond.)*, **165**, 559–568.

Jung, R. (1961) 'Neuronal Integration in the Visual Cortex and its Significance for Visual Information.' In *Sensory Communication*. Rosenblith, W. A. (Ed.). Wiley, New York.

Kuffler, S. W. (1953) Discharge patterns and functional organisation of mammalian retina. *J. Neurophysiol.*, **16**, 37–68.

Kuffler, S. W., Fitzhugh, R. and Barlow, H. B. (1957) Maintained activity in the cat's retina in light and darkness. *J. gen. Physiol.*, **40**, 683–702.

Kuffler, S. W. and Potter, D. G. (1964) Glia in the leech central nervous system: physiological properties and neuron-glia relationships. *J. Neurophysiol.*, **27**, 290–319.

Li, C-L., Ortiz-Galvin, A., Chou, S. N. and Howard, S. Y. (1960) Cortical intracellular potentials in response to stimulation of lateral geniculate body. *J. Neurophysiol.*, **23**, 592–601.

Magoun, H. W. (1935) Maintenance of the light reflex after destruction of the superior colliculus in the cat. *Amer. J. Physiol.*, **111**, 91–98.

Magoun, H. W., Atlas, D., Hare, W. K. and Ranson, S. W. (1936) The afferent path of the pupillary light reflex in the monkey. *Brain*, **59**, 234–249.

Malis, L. I. and Kruger, L. (1956) Multiple response and excitability of cat's visual cortex. *J. Neurophysiol.*, **19**, 172–186.

Maturana, H. R., Lettvin, J. Y., McCulloch, W. S. and Pitts, W. H. (1960) Anatomy and physiology of vision in the frog (Rana pipiens). *J. gen. Physiol.*, **43**, 129–176.

Michael, C. (1966) Receptive fields of directionally selective units in the optic nerve of the ground squirrel. *Science*, **132**, 1092–1095.

Michael, C. (1966) Receptive fields of opponent color units in the optic nerve of the ground squirrel. *Science*, **132**, 1095–1097.

Monnier, M. (1949) L'électro-rétinogramme de l'homme. *Electro-enceph. clin. Neurophysiol.*, **1**, 87–108.

Motokawa, K. (1963) Mechanisms for the transfer of information along visual pathways. *Int. Rev. Neurobiol.*, **5**, 121–181.

Polyak, S. L. (1941) *The Retina.* Chicago University Press, Chicago.

Polyak, S. L. (1958) *The Vertebrate Visual System.* Chicago University Press, Chicago.

Ramón y Cajal, S. (1903) Plan de estructura del tálamo óptico. *Sem. méd. (B. Aires)*, **10**, 854.

Roche, E. (Ed.) (1960) Mechanisms of vision: Caracas Symposium. *J. gen. Physiol.*, Suppl. **43**, 1–195.

Rueck, A. V. S. de and Knight, J. (Eds) (1965) *Colour Vision.* Churchill, London.

Rushton, W. A. H. (1949) The structure responsible for action potential spikes in the cat's retina. *Nature*, **164**, 743–744.

Rushton, W. A. H. (1956) The difference spectrum and the photosensitivity of rhodopsin in the living human eye. *J. Physiol. (Lond.)*, **134**, 11–29.

Scheibel, M. E. and Scheibel, A. B. (1958) 'Structural Substrates for Integrative Patterns in the Brain Stem Reticular Core.' In *Reticular Formation of the Brain.* Little, Brown, Boston.

Sechzer, J. A. and Brown, J. L. (1964) Color discrimination in the cat. *Science*, **144**, 427–429.

Spinelli, D. N., Pribram, K. H. and Weingarten, M. (1965) Centrifugal optic nerve responses evoked by auditory and somatic stimulation. *Exp. Neurol.*, **12**, 303–312.

Stone, J. and Fabian, M. (1966) Specialised receptive fields of the cat's retina. *Science*, **152**, 1277–1279.

Svaetichin, G., Laufer, M., Mitarai, G., Fatechand, R., Vallecalle, F. and Villegas, J. (1961) 'The Visual System.' In *Neurophysiology and Psychophysics.* Jung, R. and Kornhuber, H. (Eds). Springer, Berlin.

Tansley, K. (1965) *Vision in Vertebrates.* Science Paperbacks, Chapman and Hall, London.

Wald, G. (1959) 'The Photoreceptor Process in Vision.' In *Handbook of Physiology—Neurophysiology.* Vol. 1. American Physiological Society Washington.

Walls, G. L. (1942) *The Vertebrate Eye and its Adaptive Radiation.* Cranbrook Institute of Science, Michigan.

Widén, L. and Ajmone Marsan, C. (1960) Unitary analysis of the response elicited in the visual cortex of cat. *Arch. ital. Biol.*, **98**, 248–274.

Widén, L. and Ajmone Marsan, C. (1961) 'Action of Afferent and Corticofugal Impulses on Single Elements of the Dorsal Lateral Geniculate Neurones.' In *The Visual System: Neurophysiology and Psychophysics*. Jung, R., and Kornhuber, H. (Eds). Springer, Berlin.

15

Cortical Response to Peripheral Stimulation of Somatic Receptors

As is clear from the preceding chapters, nerve impulses, however initiated and wherever located, take the form of travelling action potentials, and the pathways for somatic sensation can thus be followed from the periphery, through the spinal cord, mid-brain and thalamus to the cortex. The thalamic routes to the cortex for the senses served by distance receptors have been described in Chapters 12, 13 and 14. The principal relay nuclei conveying somatic sensation are ventralis posterior medialis and ventralis posterior lateralis, which (in the anterior-posterior plane) lie in the mid-thalamus. Their names refer to the relative position in which they are found within this mass of cell groups that surround the walls of the 3rd ventricle (see Fig. 104).

The classically known pathways for somatic sensation in primates are the spinothalamic tract, the dorsal columns of the spinal cord with their first relay stations in the nuclei gracilis and cuneatus and, at a higher level, the inflow in the trigeminal nerve. In addition to these ascending pathways are the spino-bulbar tracts that feed into the reticular formation of the brain stem, and the dorsal and ventral spinocerebellar tracts. There is also evidence for abundant interconnexion with association nuclei of the thalamus by neurones with short axons. No direct afferent supply has been traced anatomically from ascending fibre systems to the association nuclei, but they have efferent projections to widespread areas of the association cortex.

The primary cortical areas for specific projection of somatic sensory impulses occupy only a small part of the cortex (in man this is principally, though not solely, the postcentral gyrus) and have a high degree of organisation for the localised receipt of impulses from the periphery. The foot is represented at the top of the postcentral convolution (of the opposite side) as it emerges from the longitudinal fissure, the trunk below this, then the arm, hand, neck and face, with the tongue and pharynx

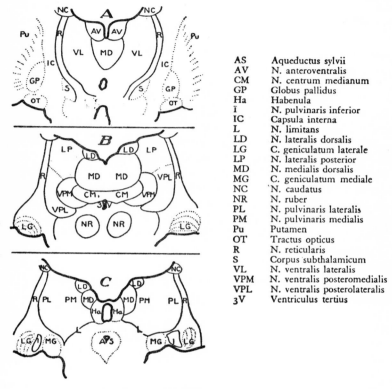

AS	Aqueductus sylvii
AV	N. anteroventralis
CM	N. centrum medianum
GP	Globus pallidus
Ha	Habenula
I	N. pulvinaris inferior
IC	Capsula interna
L	N. limitans
LD	N. lateralis dorsalis
LG	C. geniculatum laterale
LP	N. lateralis posterior
MD	N. medialis dorsalis
MG	C. geniculatum mediale
NC	N. caudatus
NR	N. ruber
PL	N. pulvinaris lateralis
PM	N. pulvinaris medialis
Pu	Putamen
OT	Tractus opticus
R	N. reticularis
S	Corpus subthalamicum
VL	N. ventralis lateralis
VPM	N. ventralis posteromedialis
VPL	N. ventralis posterolateralis
3V	Ventriculus tertius

FIG. 104. CROSS-SECTIONS OF THE THALAMUS OF THE CHIMPANZEE
IN THREE CORONAL PLANES

A, anterior thalamus; *B*, mid-thalamus; *C*, posterior thalamus.
(From Walker (1955) in *Fulton's Physiology of the Nervous System*.)

at the lowest point of the convolution (see Fig. 5). More recent work with electrodes implanted in unanaesthetised animals, as well as studies with microelectrodes has, however, revealed a greater degree of plasticity in thalamo-cortical relationships than was suggested by the initial work on animals under deep anaesthesia. The receipt of impulses from somatic sensory sources is not restricted to the primary projection areas of the cortex, for second and even third receiving areas have been located in both animals and man.

In different species the size of the cortical projection area for each part of the body varies; for example, in cats the area for the paws is proportionately large, in the dog the whiskers and lips are maximally represented, and in man and monkeys the hand is predominant. The area for the peripheral mechanism on which the animal is most dependent is the best represented in its brain.

Adrian, using a technique for recording from the surface of the brain, confirmed these localisations. He found that touching the skin produced an electrical response in the appropriate projection area. When one of the recording electrodes is on the surface of the cortical projection area and the other in the white matter of the afferent fibres from the thalamus, the first signal received is positive at the surface and negative below (in respect to any inactive area). The work of many investigators indicates that this primary evoked response, as recorded by large electrodes, is an integration of the local postsynaptic potentials of a great number of cortical neurones lying about 1 mm below the surface where the deep negativity is maximal. The initial surface positive (deep negative) potential change is followed by a longer lasting surface negative wave which is attributed to synaptic activation, i.e. EPSPs, of apical dendrites. Following these responses, which are relatively stereotyped for any given locus of the receiving cortex, there may be after-discharges of varying frequency representing a complex evocation of EPSPs and IPSPs in the cortical neurones.

For the somato-sensory cortex (in several different species) detailed maps have been made, outstanding among which are those of Woolsey and his group. In unanaesthetised animals, however, recordings from electrodes permanently implanted on the cortex reveal that the receiving areas for evoked responses are not as restricted as those found under barbiturate anaesthesia. The electrical response of the cortex has been the tool most frequently used in making these maps, but other techniques include the topical application of strychnine to the sensory cortex, by use of which Dusser de Barenne was able to detect the related skin surfaces from observation of the animal's biting and licking behaviour. In man, at operation, Penfield has mapped areas from direct verbal reports evoked by electrical stimulation of the exposed cortex.

In some early experiments Forbes and his co-workers showed that a second electrical response of the cortex to single stimula-.tion of the sciatic nerve could be detected, provided the animal

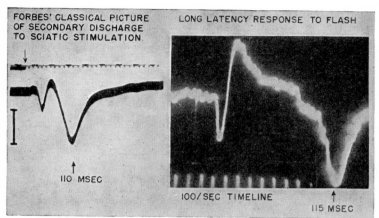

Fig. 105. *Left:* RESPONSE FROM THE CONTRALATERAL SENSORI-MOTOR CORTEX TO STIMULATION (AT THE ARROW) OF THE SCIATIC NERVE IN A CAT UNDER PENTOBARBITAL ANAESTHESIA

The record shows the primary response followed later by the larger secondary response. Vertical calibration mark 200 μV. The black dots at the top of the illustration represent 0·04-sec intervals. Negativity recorded upwards.

(From Forbes and Morison (1939) *J. Neurophysiol.*, **2**, 117.)

Right: PRIMARY AND LONG-LATENCY RESPONSE TO SINGLE FLASH RECORDED FROM VISUAL CORTEX OF A CAT UNDER PENTOBARBITAL ANAESTHESIA

(From Brazier (1958) *Reticular Formation of the Brain.* Little, Brown, Boston.)

was narcotised by a barbiturate to a sufficient depth to suppress the background electrical activity. This response was never found if the animal was anaesthetised with ether or chloroform, as these drugs block the afferent stimuli. Their records in barbiturate narcosis clearly showed an initial excursion with a latency of 8–10 msec, followed by a larger secondary discharge with a longer (and more variable) latency (30–80 msec) (see Fig. 105).

The longer latency of the secondary response cannot be explained as a delay due to vascular changes or to indirect afferent pathways through the cerebellum as it has been shown to be independent both of the sympathetic system and of the cerebello-cortical connexions. The primary response can usually be obtained only in the receiving cortex of the contralateral side, and moving the recording electrode a very few mm from the sensory area decreases the voltage very greatly, for it is a very sharply localised effect. The secondary response, unlike the primary one, appears simultaneously over most of the cortex. The difference in latency of these two responses to stimulation of the sciatic nerve is not due to their travelling to the central nervous system in fibres of different conduction rate; the threshold of excitation proves them both to be carried by the A fibres of the nerve.

Dempsey, Forbes, and Morison, in a series of experiments in which they made lesions in different parts of the brain and brain stem of cats, were able to show that the primary and secondary responses travelled by different pathways to the cortex. The primary response is carried by the classical sensory pathway to the contralateral cortex via the lateral division of the medial lemniscus and the ventro-lateral nuclei of the thalamus. The secondary response, appearing simultaneously in the cortex of both hemispheres, travels by both direct and crossing pathways. There are at least two crossed paths, one below the intercollicular level, and one above (in the anterior corpus callosum). The direct afferent path of the secondary response does not pass through the thalamus. It follows that the primary discharge cannot be the stimulus that sets off the secondary response.

A late response can also be evoked by flash in the animal under barbiturate anaesthesia (Fig. 105) and this also has been shown to reach the cortex by a route that evades the specific thalamic nucleus, i.e. the lateral geniculate. In this physiologically-evoked response in the visual system, the secondary discharge has not been found in cortex other than the visual receiving areas, but can be detected in the brain stem.

In the barbiturised animal this long-latency response to sciatic stimulation, found by Forbes, was named by him the 'secondary discharge'. From this finding it has been inferred that these impulses have travelled by an extrathalamic route distinct from the ascending reticular system, since the latter is vulnerable to barbiturate anaesthesia. The earlier difficulties of recording from moving, unanaesthetised animals during stimulation have been met by the modern computer techniques for averaging several responses and in this way emphasising the response (the 'signal') and reducing the background interference (or 'noise'). As a result, more recent work has shown that the 'Forbes secondary response' is recordable from unanaesthetised animals; the electrophysiological distinction between the two extrathalamic pathways remains. By intracellular recording from Betz cells, Purpura and his colleagues have been able to demonstrate that secondary discharges initiated by sciatic stimulation in barbiturised cats activate cortico-spinal neurons.

At the thalamic level, the electrophysiological studies of Mountcastle have revealed an extremely fine topographical projection of the body surface on to the ventrobasal nuclei of the thalamus where the main relays for somatic afferents to the cortex are to be found. Recordings with microelectrodes revealed populations of neurones in the ventrobasal thalamus which reacted maximally to localised mechanical stimulation and which signalled angle of joint rotation in specific somatotopic relation to the portion of the body receiving the peripheral stimulus via the dorsal column and medial lemniscus. In other words, a stimulus to a specific cutaneous receptive field evokes the greatest activity (i.e. highest frequency and number of short-latency discharges) in the central zone of the responding population of thalamic cells, the discharge in neighbouring neurones falling off in rate and in probability of firing.

The projections of somatic afferents from the ventrobasal thalamus to the cortex have been shown to hold the information as to nature and location of the stimulus and to carry this to specific receptive fields on the postcentral gyrus where the receiving area is considerably larger than that in the thalamic nuclei, just as the latter fields are larger than those of the dorsal column nuclei.

An important characteristic of impulse transmission in this somato-sensory afferent path through the ventrobasal thalamus is that it follows a columnar organisation. The cells in such a column reflect at each stage of the afferent path identical receptive fields in the periphery, and are activated by the same quality of stimulation of the receptors. The similarity of the initial pattern of discharge at each stage is another striking characteristic of this columnar organisation.

Mountcastle found that impulses entering the posterior thalamus via the spinothalamic tracts and projecting to the second somatic area of the cortex, did not have this markedly specific topographic (or even lateral) representation, there being

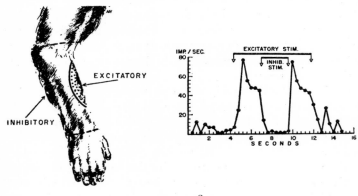

FIG. 106

An example of afferent inhibition in the somatic system of monkey. The graph is a plot of the frequency of discharge of a single cortical cell during excitatory stimulation of its own receptive field and the inhibiting action of light tactile stimulation of the large surrounding field extending from elbow to wrist.

(From Mountcastle and Powell (1959) *Johns Hopk. Hosp. Bull.*, **105**, 201.)

considerable convergence even on to individual neurones of impulses evoked by stimuli as diverse as sound and touch. He suggested therefore that the latter system, instead of coding for the nervous system the nature and location of the stimulus, signalled some other quality of sensory experience. This proposal has met its challengers who question whether the duality of function in these two systems is as clear-cut as first conceived.

Just as in the periphery where the nerves serving the centre of a receptive field fire at a higher rate than those surrounding it, so at the cortex one finds this emphasis on the topographical focus. Moreover, as Towe and Amassian first showed for the somatic system, cortical neurones in the neighbourhood of the excitatory focus are inhibited by this afferent influx (see Fig. 106). As described elsewhere in this book, the inhibitory surround is not peculiar to the somatic system but appears to be a mechanism developed for emphasis and editing of messages coming from the environment of the organism.

The introduction of microelectrode recording has brought evidence of a considerable degree of interplay at the thalamic

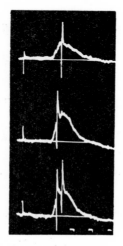

FIG. 107. SINGLE-UNIT DISCHARGES SUPERIMPOSED ON THE SLOW RESPONSES EVOKED IN THE SENSORI-MOTOR CORTEX OF THE CAT BY ULNAR NERVE STIMULATION AT THREE INTENSITIES OF VOLLEY

Note that the number of discharges and their latency changes with increasing strength of stimulus. Time line: 5-msec intervals. Negativity recorded upwards.

(From Amassian (1953) *Electroenceph. clin. Neurophysiol.*, **5**, 415.)

level, and indeed evidence for interaction between cutaneous and visceral afferents had earlier been found by Amassian. In the cortex, unit analyses of responses to peripheral stimulation have been undertaken by Li and Jasper, by Amassian and by Albe-Fessard, and since then by many others (see Fig. 107). More recently Mountcastle and his colleagues have used this technique with great success to study the response patterns of cortical neurones; Phillips was the first to succeed in obtaining intracellular recordings from pyramidal cells in the cortex of the cat, a technique now yielding increasing information about neural processes.

The study of unit responses has brought with it a change of approach to the question of how information is coded by the nervous system. The former reliance on spatial representation

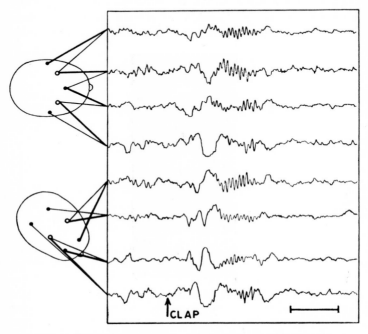

FIG. 108. THE EFFECT OF A SENSORY STIMULUS ON THE
ELECTROENCEPHALOGRAM OF MAN DURING SLEEP

The response shows a slow wave followed by a 'spindling' train of faster waves occurring bilaterally. Horizontal line indicates 1 sec.

suggested by the earlier topographical work is now complemented by the recognition of temporal characteristics, for timing, frequency and patterning of unit discharges have been shown to vary with many qualities of the stimulus, including its spatial distribution in the periphery.

In man, with the skull intact, the first example of a cortical response to sensory stimuli to be recorded was the discharge in the cortex of the sleeping subject following outside stimuli, as described by Loomis and by Davis and their colleagues, and named by them the K-complex; this was at first regarded by them as a specific auditory response but later recognised as a reaction to non-specific stimuli. An example of one of these responses during sleep is shown in Fig. 105.

A method to overcome the difficulty of detecting an evoked response against a background of continuous activity was devised by Dawson, who used a system for recording in which fifty or more successive sweeps of a cathode-ray oscillograph were superimposed in a single photograph. Exact synchrony of events was insured by a trigger circuit locked to the sweep of the oscillograph. In this way a deflection consistently following a timed impulse at a regular interval could be distinguished from randomly-occurring waves. Dawson was able by this method to detect a response in the contralateral cortex on stimulation of the ulnar nerve of man (see Fig. 109). The latency of response was longer following stimulation at the wrist than at the elbow and longer still if a nerve in the leg were stimulated. The responses were largest over the postcentral part of the brain, as far as could be judged through the unopened skull, and were restricted to quite a small area. It seems likely that these responses, which are initially surface-positive, are closely comparable to those found in the animal experiments.

A more recent design has been developed by Dawson, incorporating an automatic averaging device; another type working on the same principle, though by different electronic circuitry, was designed in collaboration with the Research Laboratory of Electronics at the Massachusetts Institute of Technology, and was used for the averaged responses illustrated in Figs 98 and 127. Yet another type of instrument for detecting small evoked responses among electroencephalographic potentials of higher amplitude has been constructed at the Lincoln Laboratories of the Massachusetts Institute of Technology. An example of how a localised response to light tapping of the hand can be recorded from electrodes on the contralateral scalp is shown in Fig. 110. Since these first pioneering developments of computer-aided analyses of biological events, many commercial designs have followed and are now on the market.

Techniques such as these, which emphasise the 'signal' at the expense of the 'noise' are of particular usefulness for studies in

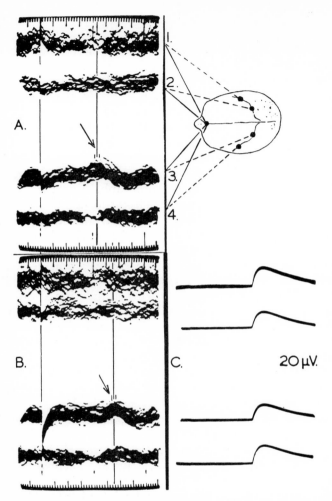

FIG. 109. CORTICAL RESPONSE TO STIMULATION OF THE RIGHT
ULNAR NERVE IN MAN

Approximately fifty successive sweeps have been superimposed in these
records. The stimulus was given in every case at the point marked by the
first vertical line. In *A* the stimulus was applied at the elbow and the
response (marked by an arrow) is seen approximately 22 msec later in the
recording from the scalp over the left sensory motor region (indifferent
electrode on the nasion). In *B* the stimulus was applied at the wrist and
the response is seen approximately 28 msec later. In *C* fifty calibration
signals of 20 μV have been superimposed. Time signals 1, 5 and 20 msec.

(From Dawson (1947) *J. Neurol. Neurosurg. Psychiat.*, **10**, 134.)

the freely moving animal. As studies progress in unanaesthetised animals with implanted electrodes it becomes clear that the responses of the brain to sensory stimuli can no longer be described in the stereotyped manner that earlier physiological work suggested, nor is the rigid distinction between sensory and motor systems so meaningful. Reasons for this great plasticity of central nervous mechanisms lie largely in the action of the reticular formation of the brain stem, a system whose influence

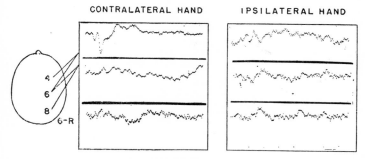

CONTRALATERAL HAND   IPSILATERAL HAND

FIG. 110. RESPONSES TO LIGHT TAPPING OF THE VOLAR SURFACE OF THE HAND, RECORDED AT THE SCALP IN A NORMAL SUBJECT

Note large evoked response in contralateral sensori-motor area and small response ipsilaterally, with a suggestion of a late wave over the association cortex. To latencies shown here, that of hammer circuit would have to be added to obtain exact time relationships. Length of sweeps: 200 msec. 90 responses averaged. M.I.T. computer (TXO).

(Brazier, Storm van Leeuwen and Molnar. Unpublished records.)

is lost in anaesthesia Moreover, inflow from various sensory modalities may interact and evoke responses in common; for example, by the use of direct-coupled amplifiers, Grey Walter has been able to demonstrate a brief diphasic wave followed by a prolonged increase in surface negativity at the vertex of the human head when the subject has been conditioned or warned to expect a second stimulus. Walter has named this the contingent negative variation. An interesting feature of this non-specific response is that if the subject is required to make a motor movement in response to the second stimulus or some purely mental decision concerning it, the negativity that has been building up during the period of expectancy is immediately terminated and, in fact, is followed by a brief surface positivity (Fig. 111).

An important influence on somatosensory inflow is exerted in the form of corticifugal control, a mechanism shared by other sensory systems. In the somaesthetic system the anatomical evidence has been provided by Kuypers who has demonstrated

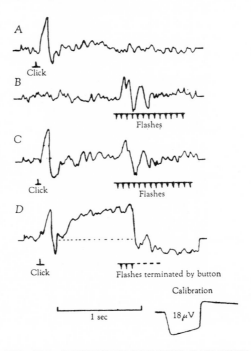

FIG. III. CONTINGENT NEGATIVE VARIATION

A, response to clicks; *B*, to flicker; *C*, clicks followed by flicker; *D*, clicks followed by flicker terminated by the subject pressing a button as instructed. Increasing negativity shown in an upward direction.
(From Walter, Cooper, Aldridge, McCallum and Winter (1964) *Nature*, **203**, 380.)

efferent fibres in the pyramidal tract from the pre- and post-central cortex and from the posterior parietal cortex which terminate in nuclei gracilis and cuneatus of the spinal cord. Electrophysiological evidence for corticifugal control in this system has been provided by the findings of Jabbur and Towe, Winter and others by unit recording in these nuclei, the majority of units being inhibited by stimulation of the sensorimotor cortex and the minority excited. Influence on units of these same nuclei can be demonstrated by stimulation of the reticular formation; in fact, participation in centrifugal modulation

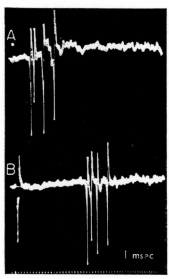

FIG. II2. RECORDINGS FROM A SINGLE NEURONE IN THE CUNEATE NUCLEUS OF A CAT

(A) when discharged centripetally by electrical stimulation of ipsilateral forepaw and (B) when discharged corticofugally by a short train of shocks applied to the ipsilateral motor cortex.

(From Jabbur and Towe (1961) in *Neural Inhibition*, Macmillan, New York. Reprinted with the permission of the Authors and the Macmillan Company.)

appears to be a characteristic of many systems within the brain, including the cerebellum.

BIBLIOGRAPHY

Adrian, E. D. (1941) Afferent discharges to the cerebral cortex from peripheral sense organs. *J. Physiol. (Lond.)*, **100,** 159–191.

Adrian, E. D. (1946) *The Physical Background of Perception.* Oxford University Press, London.

Albe-Fessard, D. and Buser, P. (1955) Activités intracellulaires recuellies dans le cortex sigmoide du chat: participation des neurones pyramidaux au 'potential évoqué' somesthésique. *J. Physiol. Path. gén,* **47,** 67–69.

Amassian, V. E. (1961) Microelectrode studies of the cerebral cortex. *Int. Rev. Neurobiol.*, **3**, 67–136.

Bard, P. (1938) Studies on the cortical representation of somatic sensibility. *Harvey Lect.*, **33**, 143–169.

Berman, A. L. (1961) Interaction of cortical responses to somatic and auditory stimuli in anterior ectosylvian gyrus of cat. *J. Neurophysiol.*, **24**, 608–620.

Berman, A. L. (1961) Overlap of somatic and auditory cortical response fields in anterior ectosylvian gyrus of cat. *J. Neurophysiol.*, **24**, 595–607.

Brazier, M. A. B. (1957) A study of the late response to flash in the cortex of the cat. *Acta physiol. pharmacol. neerl.*, **6**, 692–714.

Bremer, F. (1938) Ondes électriques de l'écorce cérébrale et influx nerveux corticifuges. *C. R. Soc. Biol. (Paris)*, **128**, 550.

Cohen, S. M. and Grundfest, H. (1954) Thalamic loci of electrical activity initiated by afferent impulses in cat. *J. Neurophysiol.*, **17**, 193–207.

Davis, H., Davis., P. A., Loomis, A. L., Harvey, E. N. and Hobart, G. (1939) Electrical reactions of the human brain to auditory stimulation during sleep. *J. Neurophysiol.*, **2**, 500–514.

Dawson, G. D. (1947) Cerebral responses to electrical stimulation of peripheral nerve in man. *J. Neurol. Neurosurg. Psychiat.*, **10**, 134–140.

Dawson, G. D. (1954) A summation technique for the detection of small evoked potentials. *Electroenceph. clin. Neurophysiol.*, **6**, 65–84.

Dempsey, E. W., Morison, R. S. and Morison, B. R. (1941) Some afferent diencephalic pathways related to cortical potentials in the cat. *Amer. J. Physiol.*, **131**, 718–731.

Derbyshire, A. J., Rempel, B., Forbes, A. and Lambert, E. F. (1936) The effects of anesthetics on action potentials in the cerebral cortex of cat. *Amer. J. Physiol.*, **116**, 577–596.

Forbes, A. and Morison, B. R. (1939) Cortical response to sensory stimulation under deep barbiturate narcosis. *J. Neurophysiol.*, **2**, 112–128.

Hagbarth, K. E. and Fex, J. (1959) Centrifugal influences in single unit activity in spinal sensory paths. *J. Neurophysiol.*, **22**, 321–358.

Holmqvist, B., Lundberg, A. and Oscarsson, O. (1960) Supraspinal inhibitory control of transmission to three ascending spinal pathways influenced by the flexion reflex afferents. *Arch. ital. Biol.*, **98**, 60–80.

Holmqvist, B., Lundberg, A. and Oscarsson, O. (1960) A supraspinal control system monosynaptically connected with an ascending spinal pathway. *Arch. ital. Biol.*, **68**, 402–422.

Jabbur, S. J. and Towe, A. L. (1961) Cortical excitation of neurons in dorsal column nuclei of cat, including an analysis of pathways. *J. Neurophysiol.*, **24**, 499–509.

Kuypers, H. G. J. M. (1960) Central cortical projections to motor and somatosensory cell groups. *Brain*, **83**, 161–184.

Li, C. L. and Jasper, H. (1953) Microelectrode studies of the electrical activity of the cerebral cortex in the cat. *J. Physiol.* (*Lond.*), **121**, 117–140.

Lundberg, A. and Oscarsson, O. (1962) Two ascending spinal pathways in the ventral part of the cord. *Acta physiol. scand.*, **54**, 270–286.

Magoun, H. W. and McKinley, W. A. (1942) The termination of ascending trigeminal and spinal tracts in the thalamus of the cat. *Amer. J. Physiol.*, **137**, 409–416.

Marshall, W. H., Woolsey, C. N. and Bard, P. (1941) Representation of tactile sensibility in the monkey's cortex as indicated by cortical potentials. *J. Neurophysiol.*, **4**, 1–24.

Morison, R., Dempsey, E. W. and Morison, B. (1941) On the propagation of certain cortical potentials. *Amer. J. Physiol.*, **131**, 744–751.

Mountcastle, V. B. (1961) 'Duality of function in the somatic afferent system.' In *Brain and Behavior*. Brazier, M. A. B. (Ed.) Vol. I. American Institute of Biological Science, Washington.

Mountcastle, V. B. (1957) Modality and topographic properties of single neurons of cat's somatic sensory cortex. *J. Neurophysiol.*, **20**, 408–434.

Mountcastle, V. B., Davies, P. W. and Berman, A. L. (1957) Response properties of neurons of cat's somatic sensory cortex to peripheral stimuli. *J. Neurophysiol.*, **20**, 374–407.

Mountcastle, V. B. and Henneman, E. (1952) The representation of tactile sensibility in the thalamus of the monkey. *J. comp. Neurol.*, **97**, 409–440.

Mountcastle, V. B., Poggio, G. F. and Werner, G. (1963) The relation of thalamic cell response to peripheral stimuli varied over an intensive continuum. *J. Neurophysiol.*, **26**, 807–834.

Penfield, W. (1947) Some observations on the cerebral cortex of man. *Proc. roy. Soc. B.*, **134**, 329.

Perl, E. R. (1963) Somatosensory mechanisms. *Ann. Rev. Physiol.*, **25**, 459–492.

Phillips, C. G. (1956) Intracellular records from Betz cells in the cat. *Quart. J. exp. Physiol.*, **41**, 58–69.

Purpura, D. P., Cohen, B. and Marini, G. (1961) Generalised neocortical responses and corticospinal neuron activity. *Science*, **134**, 729–730.

Renshaw, B., Forbes, A. and Morison, B. R. (1940) Activity of the isocortex and hippocampus: electrical studies with microelectrodes. *J. Neurophysiol.*, **3**, 74–105.

Ruch, T. C., Patton, H. D. and Amassian, V. E. (1952) Topographical and functional determinants of cortical localisation patterns. *Res. Publ. Ass. nerv. ment. Dis.*, **30**, 403–429.

Towe, A. L. and Amassian, V. E. (1958) Patterns of activity in single cortical units following stimulation of the digits in monkeys. *J. Neurophysiol.*, **21**, 292–311.

Walter, W. G., Cooper, R., Aldridge, V. J., McCallum, W. C. and Winter, A. L. (1964) Contingent negative variation: an electric sign of sensori-motor association and expectancy in the human brain. *Nature*, **203**, 380–384.

Werner, G. and Mountcastle, V. B. (1965) Neural activity in mechano-receptive cutaneous afferents: stimulus-response relations, Weber functions, and information transmission. *J. Neurophysiol.*, **28**, 359–397.

Winter, D. L. (1965) N. Gracilis of cat. Functional organisation and corticifugal effects. *J. Neurophysiol.*, **28**, 48–70.

Woolsey, C. N. (1952) 'Patterns of localisation in sensory and motor areas of the cerebral cortex.' In *The Biology of Mental Health*. Hoeber, New York.

16

The Electrical Activity of the Brain

THE detection of the electrical changes evoked in the cortex by stimulation of sensory systems is always made difficult in the unanaesthetised animal by the presence of continuous electrical activity at the cortex. These persistent fluctuating potentials were discovered in 1875 by Caton who described them as 'feeble currents of the brain'. The amplitude of these electrical oscillations being so low (i.e. in the order of microvolts) Caton's discovery of them is all the more remarkable in that it was made about half a century before electronic amplification became available in the biological laboratory.

By the end of the nineteenth century several laboratories in Poland and Russia had confirmed Caton's findings. In the early years of this century Neminski in Russia defined in dogs two principal frequency ranges which later were also found in man, and which are known as alpha and beta activity. The alpha rhythm (which is described for man in the next chapter), being the most prominent, was the first to receive intensive exploration. This persistent background activity, present even in the apparent absence of any specifically directed peripheral stimulus, has been extensively studied, and this branch of electrophysiology has earned a name of its own: electroencephalography.

One of the least understood of all the properties of nerve cells is their apparent tendency, when in aggregates, to produce extracellular current-flows of a rhythmic nature. This tendency is very commonly referred to as 'spontaneous' activity but, as applied here, this word can have no very clear meaning for a physiologist. The impetus could come to the nerve cells by many agents: change in membrane impedance, intra- and extra-cellular chemical change, simple synaptic transmission, facilitation by random bombardment, facilitation by rhythmic bombardment, facilitation by impulses circulating in closed circuits, spread of extrinsic currents from adjacent active neurones and electrotonic spread of the type found by Barron and Matthews in the spinal cord. All these factors influence the excitability of neurones and any or all may contribute to the production of a rhythmic current flow from a group of nerve cells.

In the first half of this century nerve physiology was dominated by the 'all-or-nothing' law and by discoveries that were being made in axonology. It naturally followed that attempts to explain the comparatively slow potential changes of the brain should first be made in terms of axon spikes. The brief, staccato-like action potentials of the familiar nerve impulse have, however, a duration of less than 1 msec (in contrast to the 100-msec duration of the alpha wave), so that very many of them, slightly asynchronous in their discharge, would be needed to give the envelope of one alpha wave.

It will be noticed that any concept that considered the axon spike as the building block of the cortical wave implied neuronal activity in the form of a discharge, although all the empirical observations of the alpha wave, in both man and animals, pointed to its being a phenomenon not of action, but of 'the engine when idling', i.e. of the brain at rest (though not asleep). Early in the development of this branch of electrophysiology, Bremer suggested that the oscillating potentials were the sign of 'tonus' in the cortex, indicators of fluctuation in excitability rather than of discharge. This concept, that normal electroencephalographic potentials are concomitants of the excitability changes of cortical neurones, is basic to today's thinking.

The patent inadequacy of axonology to provide the explanation of brain waves led investigators to propose next that the cell bodies of cortical neurones might be the source, but they were still thinking in terms of conducted discharges and these too were awkwardly short in duration (2 to 3 msec) to account for the 10 per second oscillations.

Looking back more than thirty years across the accumulation of modern findings, one sees that it was Forbes who, in 1936, first suggested to physiologists that they should recognise that spike potentials, whether originating from axons or from soma, were fundamentally different in character from slow waves, and that these two distinct categories of bioelectric phenomena occurred in neurones.

Some years were to pass before this distinction took root in neurophysiology and it was not until the clear demonstration of graded potentials in dendrites that the attention of electro-encephalographers was caught.

In 1936 the American Physiological Society heard the results of the first successful microelectrode recordings from cortical cells described by Forbes, and two years later microelectrode recordings from hippocampal cells were reported by his colleague Renshaw. Their conclusions were that 'all evidence indicates that the slow waves are not the summations of numbers of axon-like spikes'. That the work of this team laid the groundwork for today's understanding of brain waves becomes apparent when one reads the fuller account of their pioneer work on extracellular unit potentials published in 1940. Their studies pinpointed the slow potential to the neighbourhood of the synapse and dissociated it from the spike discharge.

When linked with the growing realisation of the role of dendrites, the pieces of the jig-saw puzzle began to fall into place. Lorente de Nó, in 1934, had emphasised that dendrites had the characteristic property of never becoming refractory. Multiple incoming stimuli could give a summated response. This finding has been consistently confirmed by subsequent workers.

If the oscillating potentials recorded from the scalp originate in cortical neurones they must be derived from neurones whose component units are uniformly oriented, for were they randomly distributed their potential fields would tend to cancel each other. One of the outstanding contributions that the physiologist with his microelectrode has made in recent years is the demonstration that all parts of a neurone do not have the same electrical characteristics. Not only are the time characteristics of the spike discharge greatly different for the cell body, the axon and the dendrite respectively, but the recovery rates after a discharge are vastly different. This means that activity in any part of a cell or its processes sets up a flow of extracellular current between the rapidly repolarising areas of membrane and the more slowly recovering parts. Some discussion of these contrasting properties of the different parts of a neurone has already been given in Chapter 3.

In the cortex, for the extracellular current flows to reach a density that can be recorded at the scalp, they must be closely massed and flowing predominantly in the same direction. A field of current dense enough to meet these requirements, from structures geometrically oriented so that the voltage gradients they present at the cortex could be sufficiently steep, is found

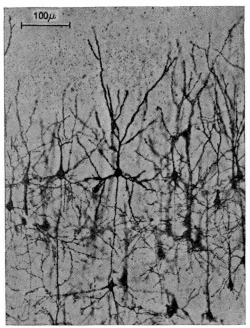

FIG. 113. PHOTOGRAPH OF A SECTION THROUGH THE VISUAL CORTEX OF A CAT SHOWING PYRAMIDAL CELLS WITH THEIR APICAL DENDRITES EXTENDING UPWARDS TOWARDS THE CORTEX. GOLGI-COX STAIN
(From Sholl (1953) *J. Anat. (Lond.)*, **87**, 387.)

in the radially-orientated apical shafts of the pyramidal cells, reaching up and branching towards the cortical surface (see Figs. 113, 114). Moreover, these long dendritic processes are known to have electrical characteristics radically different from those of their cells and axons and thus, with their extensive area of membrane, constitute a powerful source of extracellular current. It should be noted, however, that on anatomical grounds this is a vast oversimplification, for the cell structure and layering of the cortex, especially in regions other than the visual receiving area (where, granted, the alpha rhythm is most prominent) is of a complexity that defies an analysis such as this

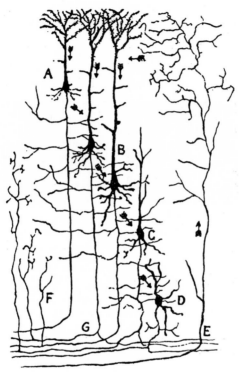

FIG. 114. RAMÓN Y CAJAL'S DRAWING OF PYRAMIDAL CELLS (*A* AND *B*) WITH APICAL DENDRITES REACHING TO THE CORTICAL SURFACE

The afferent fibre, *E*, is shown sending off branches at all levels within the cortex, and an arrow in the upper layers indicates axo-dendritic synapsis on to apical dendrites.

(From Ramón y Cajal (1894) *Les Nouvelles Idées sur la Structure du Système nerveux chez l'Homme et chez les Vertébrés.* Reiwald, Paris.)

which ignores other cellular components whose orientation is less conspicuous. Nevertheless, the evidence, although inferential, for linking the potentials of apical dendrites to the electro-encephalogram is the best at hand at present. No other structures with sufficient membrane surface in the required orientation for adequate current density have yet been suggested.

With the recognition of the characteristics of postsynaptic potentials (as described earlier in this book) having a long duration of their decay (80 to 100 sec), attention finally turned away from axon or cell discharges to these slow, graded responses as being the building blocks of brain waves.

Once it became logical to implicate cortical dendrites in the mechanism of brain waves it became necessary to establish more firmly the electrical characteristics of these structures, and

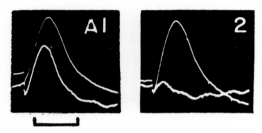

FIG. 115. SURFACE EVOKED POTENTIALS

A1: Surface negative responses of the cerebral cortex of a cat recorded at a site 1 mm distant from the stimulus location where pulses 0·1 msec in duration were applied.   Top trace from a silver ball electrode; lower trace from a 100η wire electrode. Both electrodes on the cortical surface. 2: Wire electrode (second trace) lowered to 0·4 mm below surface. Time line: 20 msec.

(From Purpura (1957) *Science*, **125**, 1200).

this has largely been effected by studying the potential changes evoked by electrical stimulation of the cortical surface (Fig. 115).

This is a laboratory technique which, although having no physiological counterpart, has contributed significantly to the understanding of dendritic potentials. As shown long ago by Adrian, such a stimulus evokes a slow potential change. This response, which is not all-or-nothing in character but proportional to the strength of the stimulus, can be recorded from a region around the point where the stimulus is applied. These superficial cortical responses have received considerable study from several workers and outstandingly by Purpura, who has presented the evidence for assigning them to postsynaptic potentials of superficially located dendrites. Purpura's study of them in relation to growth of dendrites in immature animals leads him to the conclusion that the spread of activity to regions distant from the stimulus point is by conduction in horizontal fibres in the molecular layer of the cortex.

The many cells responsible for adding their activity in such a way as to produce waves of the amplitude of alpha waves must have their major electrical characteristics in common. In a population of dendrites this would necessitate some regulatory mechanism for the summation of hyperpolarising and depolarising postsynaptic potentials in the complex of their parent neurones. Clarification of this problem obviously cannot come from electrodes recording extracellularly from the cortical surface, for such electrodes average, not only from neuronal activity surrounding them in two-dimensional space, but also summate electrical activity from a few millimetres below the surface. They cannot therefore differentiate between an excitatory postsynaptic potential at the surface and an inhibitory postsynaptic potential in deeper layers: both will present apparent negativity at the surface. Such a differentiation can, however, be made by the application of certain pharmacological agents such as strychnine which abolishes the intracellular IPSPs which are however resistant to gamma amino butyric acid, an agent which has a markedly depressing effect on EPSPs.

Thus, once the electrical properties of cortical dendrites had been established, the problem still remained as to how to account for the remarkable rhythmicity of cortical activity.

Much early work was directed towards a search for a pacemaker mechanism responsible for the rhythmic activity of groups of neurones in such a way that they summate smoothly and rhythmically, and for the factor which could hold them to this beat. It was recognised that these mechanisms might be essentially either chemical, neuronal or directly electrotonic in nature, or perhaps all three, though electrotonic conduction between neurones, sufficiently common in fish, is evidently rare in mammalian species. A chemical pacemaker was postulated by those who held that the brain waves were due to the continuous building up of potentials by metabolism in nerve cells; the potentials would discharge every time a critical level was reached (in a manner comparable to a relaxation oscillator). This hypothesis was formulated by Hoagland at a time when attention was mainly directed towards cell discharge as the unit component of the alpha wave. His work on the increase in the rate of the alpha rhythm with temperature rise and with other stimulators of metabolism supported the hypothesis that relative frequency changes under specific conditions were related to change in rate of cell metabolism, but did not define the bio-electric origin of the waves.

Attention was turned to the role of thalamic neurones in evoking rhythmic activity in the cortex by the work of Bremer, and was strikingly demonstrated in 1941 by Adrian who showed that a single afferent volley to a peripheral nerve produced rhythmical waves in the receiving cortex and in the radiations from the specific thalamic relay nucleus. Since then confirmation has come from many workers as well as in relation to other thalamic relays including the lateral and medial geniculate nuclei. The classic studies of Morison and Dempsey, published in the 1940s, confirmed the dependence of EEG activity on thalamo-cortical relationships.

In more modern times, intracellular recordings have led to the view that an alternation of excitation and post-excitatory inhibition in thalamic neurones may be the basis for the rhythmic synchronisation of cortical neurones, Purpura and others having demonstrated the long duration of IPSPs of thalamic neurones with their damping effect on spontaneous and evoked discharges.

When unit recordings are made from cortical cells an interruption of the on-going rhythmic discharge follows any brief excitation; intracellular exploration by Albe-Fessard and her collaborators have shown these interruptions to coincide with a wave of long duration (100 to 200 msec), the inside of the cell being negative to the outside. As these waves of long duration also occur in the absence of stimulation they therefore cannot be regarded as merely a post-excitatory phase dependent on an afferent stimulus.

Thus, evidence certainly exists for active inhibitory mechanisms in the cortex. Some time ago Li demonstrated that pyramidal cell discharges can be arrested by cortical or thalamic volleys and further evidence has come from other workers. Most of these have envisaged the inhibitory influences being exerted through an interneurone (as generally accepted for the spinal cord). It has also been suggested that the inhibition may be located in the presynaptic fibres in a manner analogous to that suggested by Eccles for presynaptic inhibition in the spinal cord. One of the characteristics of presynaptic inhibition, as defined in the spinal cord, is its long duration, and this has been found by Li, Creutzfeldt and others in cortical cells following cortical and subcortical stimuli. Jung has therefore suggested that postsynaptic potentials of apical dendrites may not be the only source of brain waves, another being the depolarisation of inhibition in presynaptic fibres.

At the time of writing, the exploration of the role of thalamic regulation of the EEG is one of the most active fields of investigation and, doubtless, critical evidence will emerge from these studies which will define whether the gating action of long-duration inhibitory potentials operates through recurrent collaterals from thalamo-cortical neurones (as suggested by Eccles), or whether the rhythmic inhibition may not come from synaptic interaction between neurones in specific and nonspecific thalamic nuclei including those that receive input from the caudate and from the cerebellum (as proposed by Purpura). The question of the necessity for postulating an inhibitory interneurone has yet to be resolved definitively.

Several attempts have been made to establish the relationships between EEG activity and the discharges of single cortical cells. Consistent with the hypothesis outlined above is the early finding of Li and Jasper that the brief spike discharges of cell units in the cortex as recorded by microelectrodes seemed unrelated to the slow waves in the resting rhythm of the cat.

In 1940, Renshaw, Forbes and Morison, the first physiologists to record unit potentials from the brain, could find no relation between the slow waves recordable from the hippocampal surface and unit discharges from the pyramidal cells. Since those days the pyramidal cells of the hippocampus have been extensively explored by Green and others as neurones analogous to the Betz cells of the neocortex but with markedly less complexity of interconnection. The question of the relationship of unit discharges to rhythmic activity in hippocampal cells was explored by Green and Machne, who were unable to establish any exact phase relation of the spike discharge to the rhythmic activity at any depth of the hippocampal cortex.

Brookhart and his associates working in the cerebellum (which has a characteristic rhythm of 200 to 300/sec) found these waves to be independent of the unitary discharge of cells within the cerebellar cortex. It may be noted in passing that both the pyramidal cells of the hippocampus and the Purkinje cells of the cerebellum have dendritic trees with a large expanse of membrane surface. It was Jasper's conclusion from his microelectrode studies that the slow waves of the alpha rhythm

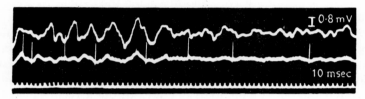

FIG. 116. UNITARY SPIKE DISCHARGES WITHOUT CLEAR PHASE RELATIONSHIP TO THE ALPHA WAVES AND CONTINUING LONGER THAN THE ALPHA BURST (CAT)

The upper trace was recorded with a large electrode on the cortical surface and a long time constant, the lower trace with a microelectrode at a depth of 1,600 μ below the surface and a short time constant. Negativity recorded upwards.

(From Li and Jasper (1953) *J. Physiol. (Lond.)*, **121**, 117.)

behaved as though they represented synaptic potentials, independent of neuronal cell discharge, though related in a complex manner to the excitability of cortical cells (Fig. 116).

The linking of EEG waves to excitability changes in the cortex was strongly suggested by the early finding of Adrian and Moruzzi that these waves bore a relation to the efferent outflow as recorded from the pyramidal tract.

With the recognition that the EEG waves are summations of excitatory and inhibitory postsynaptic potentials generated at many different levels in the cortex, it is not surprising that extracellularly placed microelectrodes may pick up large fields of extracellular current flows while not necessarily being optimally positioned near the spike generating membrane of any one cell. Thus a negative finding cannot provide definitive evidence, and those cases where some phase relationship has been found are of great interest. As Pollen, Marsan and others have shown, closer relationships between unit discharge and slow wave is found in conditions where the EEG is itself exhibiting marked rhythmicity. This may be occurring normally, as in a 'spindle burst' or be induced by drugs, or by disease states as, for example, in the 3 per second discharges of petit mal epilepsy (described in Chapter 19) or in the tremor of Parkinsonism in man.

As research has progressed on cortical activity, as represented by the EEG, the importance of subcortical mechanisms has now received full recognition. The influence of the mesencephalic brain stem and the thalamic reticular system on the electrical activity of the cortex forms the subject of the next chapter.

BIBLIOGRAPHY

Adrian, E. D. (1941) Afferent discharges to the cerebral cortex from peripheral sense organs. *J. Physiol.*, **100**, 159–191.

Adrian, E. D. (1947) General principles of nervous activity. *Brain*, **70**, 1–17.

Adrian, E. D. and Moruzzi, G. (1939) Impulses in the pyramidal tract. *J. Physiol. (Lond.)*, **97**, 153–199.

Albe-Fessard, D. (1960) Sur l'origine des ondes lentes observées en dérivation intracellulaire dans diverse structures cérébrales. *C. R. Soc. Biol. (Paris)*, **154**, 11–16.

Andersen, P. (1966) 'Rhythmic 10/sec activity in the thalamus.' In *The Thalamus*. Purpura, D. P. and Yahr, M. D. (Eds). Columbia University Press, New York.

Andersen, P., Andersson, S. A. and Lømo, T. (1966) Patterns of spontaneous activity within various thalamic nuclei. *Nature*, **211**, 888–889.

Andersen, P. and Eccles, J. C. (1962) Inhibitory phasing of neuronal discharge. *Nature*, **196**, 645–647.

Bishop, G. H. (1956) The natural history of the nerve impulse. *Physiol. Rev.*, **36**, 376–399.

Bremer, F. (1938) *L'Activité Électrique de l'Écorce Cérébrale.* Hermann, Paris.

Caton, R. (1875) The electrical currents of the brain. *Brit. med. J.*, **ii**, 278.

Clare, M. H. and Bishop, G. H. (1955) Properties of dendrites: apical dendrites of the cortex. *Electroenceph. clin. Neurophysiol.*, **7**, 85–98.

Creutzfeldt, O. D., Lux, H. D. and Watanabe, S. (1966) 'Electrophysiology of cortical nerve cells.' In *The Thalamus*. Purpura,

D. P. and Yahr, M. D. (Eds). Columbia University Press, New York.

Dempsey, E. W. and Morison, R. S. (1943) The electrical activity of a thalamocortical relay system. *Amer. J. Physiol.*, **138**, 283–296, 297–308.

Eccles, J. C. (1951) Interpretation of action potentials evoked in the cerebral cortex. *Electroenceph. clin. Neurophysiol.*, **3**, 449–464.

Forbes, A., Renshaw, B. and Rempel, B. (1937) Units of electrical activity in the cerebral cortex. *Amer. J. Physiol.*, **119**, 309–310.

Freeman, W. J. (1963) The electrical activity of a primary sensory cortex: analysis of EEG waves. *Int. Rev. Neurobiol.*, **5**, 53–119.

Fromm, G. H. and Bond, H. W. (1964) Slow changes in the electrocorticogram and the activity of cortical neurons. *Electroenceph. clin. Neurophysiol.*, **17**, 520–523.

Frost, J. D. and Goll, A. (1966) Computer determination of relationships between EEG activity and single unit discharges in isolated cerebral cortex. *Exp. Neurol.*, **14**, 506–519.

Green, J. D. and Machne, X. (1955) Unit activity of rabbit hippocampus. *Amer. J. Physiol.*, **181**, 219–224.

Hoagland, H. (1936) Pacemakers of human brain waves in normals and in general paretics. *Amer. J. Physiol.*, **116**, 604.

Jung, R. (1963) 'Central inhibitory phenomena.' In *Progress in Brain Research*. Vol. I. Moruzzi, G., Fessard, A. and Jasper, H. H. (Eds). Elsevier, Amsterdam.

Klee, M. R., Offenlock, K. and Tigges, J. (1965) Cross-correlation analysis of electroencephalographic potentials and slow membrane transients. *Science*, **147**, 519–521.

Krnjevic, K., Randić, M. and Straughan, D. W. (1966) An inhibitory process in the cerebral cortex. *J. Physiol. (Lond.)*, **184**, 16–48, 49–77, 78–105.

Li, Ch-L. (1956) The inhibitory effect of stimulation of a thalamic nucleus on neuronal activity in the motor cortex. *J. Physiol. (Lond.)*, **133**, 40–53.

Li, Ch-L. and Jasper, H. (1953) Microelectrode studies of the electrical activity of the cerebral cortex in the cat. *J. Physiol. (Lond.)*, **121**, 117–140.

Lorente de Nó, R. (1934) Studies on the structure of the cerebral cortex. *J. Psychol. Neurol. (Lpz.)*, **46**, 113–177.

Martin, A. R. and Branch, C. L. (1958) Spontaneous activity of Betz cells in cats with midbrain lesions. *J. Neurophysiol.*, **21**, 368–390.

Moruzzi, G. and Magoun, H. W. (1949) Brain stem reticular formation and activation of the EEG. *Electroenceph. clin. Neurophysiol.*, **1**, 455–473.

Pollen, D. and Sie, P. G. (1964) Analysis of thalamically induced wave and spike by modification in cortical excitability. *Electroenceph. clin. Neurophysiol.*, **17**, 154–163.

Pollen, D. A. and Ajmone Marsan, C. (1965) Cortical inhibitory postsynaptic potentials and strychninisation. *J. Neurophysiol.*, **28**, 432–458.

Purpura, D. P. (1959) Nature of electrocortical potentials and synaptic organisations in cerebral and cerebellar cortex. *Int. Rev. Neurobiol.*, **1**, 47–163.

Purpura, D. P. and Cohen, B. (1962) Intracellular recording from thalamic neurons during recruiting responses. *J. Neurophysiol.*, **25**, 621–635.

Purpura, D. P., Frigyesi, T. L., McMurtry, J. G. and Scarff, T. (1966) 'Synaptic mechanisms in thalamic regulation of cerebello-cortical projection activity.' In *The Thalamus*. Purpura, D. P. and Yahr, M. D. (Eds). Columbia University Press, New York.

Purpura, D. P. and Shofer, R. J. (1963) Intracellular recording from thalamic neurons during reticulo-cortical activation. *J. Neurophysiol.*, **26**, 494–505.

Renshaw, B., Forbes, A. and Drury, C. (1938) Electrical activity recorded with microelectrodes from the hippocampus. *Amer. J. Physiol.*, **123**, 169–170.

Renshaw, B., Forbes, A. and Morison, B. R. (1940) Activity of isocortex and hippocampus: electrical studies with micro-electrodes. *J. Neurophysiol.*, **3**, 74–105.

Walter, W. G. (1950) The functions of electrical rhythms in the brain. *J. ment. Sci.*, **96**, 1–31.

17

The Electrical Activity of the Brain Stem and Thalamic Reticular Systems

In the brain stem, among the long ascending and descending fibre tracts that pass through it, lie many nuclei, the nuclei for the cranial nerves being the most prominent. But in addition to the latter there is a central network of neural tissue containing cells which give rise to longitudinal fibres of considerable length, running both rostrally and caudally (Fig. 117). Branching collaterals from the axons together with prolific dendritic ramifications from the cell bodies, mostly at right angles to the longitudinal axis, form what Herrick described as 'a web of tissue'. And because of its net-like structure this crowded mesh is known as the reticular formation of the brain stem.

The reticular formation extends through the central core of the bulb, pons and mid-brain, resembling in some ways a rostral continuation of the grey matter that extends throughout the spinal cord. Functionally, and to a cetain degree topographically, two main influences may be differentiated at the level of the brain stem: a descending system, modulating spinal activity by inhibitory and facilitatory influences, and an ascending system of powerful influence over the hypothalamus, thalamus, the neocortex, and the older rhinencephalic structures.

The Descending System. In 1944 Magoun demonstrated that electrical stimulation of the ventromedial part of the bulbar reticular formation decreases or abolishes flexor and extensor reflexes and motor activity evoked by cortical stimulation in the cat anaesthetised with chloralose. In an animal with decerebrate rigidity, its extended limbs collapse into flaccidity. Evidence that this strong inhibitory action on motion is not seen on stimulation in the unanaesthetised animal suggests that these descending effects are apparently inhibited by a return feedback control exerted by the cortex on the reticular neurones.

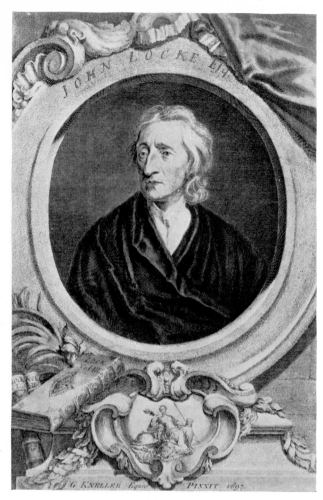

PLATE V

John Locke (1632–1704)

whose theory of knowledge derived all ideas from sensation
and perception.

'It is about these impressions made on our senses by outward objects, that
the mind seems first to employ itself, in such operations as we call perception,
remembering, consideration, reasoning . . .' (*Essay Concerning Humane Understanding*, 1690)

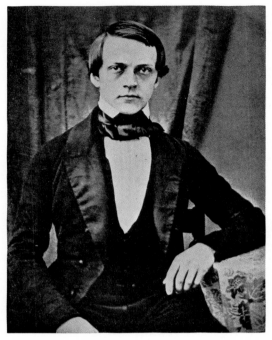

PLATE VI

Hermann von Helmholtz (1821–1894)

Brilliant physiologist and physicist, formulator of the Law of Conservation
of Energy, master in the field of optics, and author of the theory of hearing
from which all modern theories of resonance are derived.

This is certainly strongly indicated in the case of the facilitatory system (described below) by the experiments of Hugelin and Bonvallet. The descending inhibitory path is rapidly conducting and in the cord its fibres run down mostly in the ventral part of the lateral funiculus crossing at lower levels to act on

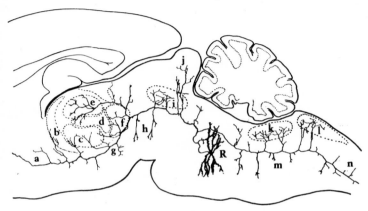

FIG. 117. A SAGITTAL SECTION OF TWO-DAY RAT SHOWING A SINGLE LARGE RETICULAR NEURONE OF THE NUCLEUS GIGANTOCELLULARIS OF THE MEDULLA

The large cell emits an axon which bifurcates into caudal and rostral-running segments. The caudal segment projects upon spinal proprio-neurones and motor neurones. The rostral segment extends into both dorsal and ventral subthalamus. Some branches may project monosynaptically upon cortex as suggested by Golgi anatomy studies and the experiments of Magni and Willis (1964) *Arch. ital. Biol.*, **102**, 418. Numerous collaterals are given off by both segments *en route* through the neuraxis. Areas innervated include (*a*) basal forebrain; (*b*) nucleus reticularis thalami; (*c*) commissural nuclei of medial thalamus; (*d*) thalamic intralaminar system; (*e*) dorso-medial nucleus; (*f*) centromedianparafascicular complex; (*g*) zona incerta; (*h*) mesencephalic tegmentum; (*i*) nuclei of 3rd and 4th cranial nerves; (*j*) inferior colliculus; (*k*) nucleus of 12th cranial nerve; (*l*) nucleus gracilis; (*m*) medullary reticular formation; (*n*) ventral half of spinal cord.

(By courtesy of Scheibel and Scheibel. Unpublished.)

spinal interneurones. Stimulation through microelectrodes in the intermediate internuncial pool in the lower cord has been shown to inhibit the knee jerk and this presumably forms the last stage of the process.

In cats and monkeys under chloralose anaesthesia, Rhines and Magoun found a descending facilitatory system that could be activated at levels in the brain stem above the bulb and extending as far forward as the subthalamus, hypothalamus and basal parts of the thalamus itself. The descending path, like that of the inhibitory system, is of low threshold for stimulation and is rapidly conducting, passing down the lateral funiculus in the cord, rather more dorsally than the inhibitory system fibres but with some overlap. The facilitating influence

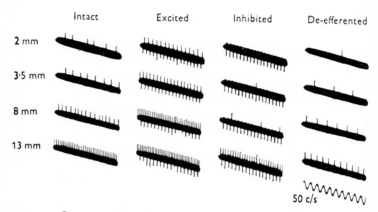

FIG. 118. RECORDINGS FROM SINGLE AFFERENT FIBRES FROM A MUSCLE SPINDLE AT 4° OF STRETCH (AS NOTED IN mm TO THE LEFT OF THE OSCILLOGRAPHIC TRACES)

Columns from left to right show: the intact control state; the increase in rate of discharge on stimulation of the contralateral inferior colliculus; the decrease on stimulation of the contralateral internal capsule; and the effect of cutting the efferent supply to the spindle. Nerve discharges recorded in an upward direction, stimulus pulses downwards.

(From Eldred, Granit and Merton (1953) *J. Physiol.* (*Lond.*), **122**, 498.)

on spinal motor neurones, partially directly but more importantly through interneurones, has been elucidated by the work of Lloyd.

In 1949 Snider and Magoun demonstrated the influence of the cerebellum on reticulo-spinal mechanisms, and since then Moruzzi and his colleagues at Pisa have studied these relationships in great detail. Evidence for reticular control has also been found to be mediated partially through the caudate nucleus. In the physiological, unanaesthetised animal, therefore, it seems likely that the stimulating influence that maintains the reticulo-spinal inhibitory and facilitatory effects at optimal level for the organism comes from the cortex and cerebellum.

Lloyd has made the suggestion that this extrapyramidal, cortico-reticulo-spinal route, being rapidly conducting, provides a mechanism by which the stage can be set in the cord for arrival of the more directly, but more slowly conducted pyramidal discharges.

In a previous chapter (Chapter 10, page 129) the reflex control of muscle spindles by gamma efferent fibres was described. From Granit's laboratory has come the evidence that this regulatory feedback is also strongly influenced by higher centres. Stimulation of a point in the contralateral inferior colliculus was found by Eldred, Granit and Merton to increase the rapidity of firing in single fibres from muscle spindles, whereas stimulation at a point in the contralateral internal capsule decreased the rate of discharge or abolished it in a degree comparable to that effected by cutting the efferent supply (see Fig. 118).

The Ascending Reticular Activating System. In 1935 Bremer discovered that in the cat, transection of the brain stem at the intercollicular level below the nucleus of the 3rd nerve (see Fig. 119) results in an animal that cannot be aroused by sensory stimulation and that has the EEG and eye signs of sleep. The EEG signs are slow waves of high amplitude, and the eye sign is a narrowed pupil. Since this transection isolates the cerebrum from the rest of the brain and brain stem Bremer named this preparation the *'cerveau isolé'*. A cut lower down (at the first cervical segment) does not have this effect, the EEG and eye signs remaining those of an awake cat. The latter preparation isolates the whole brain and brain stem from the spinal cord and therefore Bremer named it the *'encéphale isolé'*. He concluded that afferent inflow, interrupted by the higher transection, was vital to the maintenance of the waking state, the usual level of sensory influx in the two surviving sensory nerves, olfactory and optic, being generally insufficient, although extremely strong olfactory stimulation can evoke EEG arousal patterns in such an animal.

In 1949 Moruzzi and Magoun discovered that maintenance of wakefulness does not depend on inflow to the cortex carried by the specific sensory radiations, but on impulses travelling in a hitherto undemonstrated extralemniscal sensory system. Their electrophysiological work established the existence of sensory afferent routes to the cortex additional to the classical specific pathways. They named these the *ascending reticular activating system.*

Their initial discovery was that electrical stimulation of the reticular system (with optimal frequency of 100 to 300/sec)

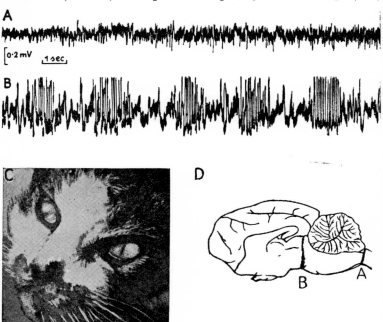

FIG. 119. ELECTROCORTICOGRAMS OF A CAT

A: Activity typical of the alert state in an *encéphale isolé* preparation
(transection made at *A* in section *D*).

B: The spindling activity recorded from the *cerveau isolé* preparation
(transection made at *B* in section *D*). The slit pupil of the latter preparation, similar to that of a sleeping cat, is seen in section *C*.

(From Bremer (1937) *Bull. Acad. roy. Méd. Belg.*, **2**, 68.)

changes the sleep-like slow waves of high voltage of an animal under chloralosane anaesthesia, or that of an *encéphale isolé* preparation, to the fast activity of low amplitude typical of the alert waking state (see Fig. 120). This change in the EEG long outlasts the duration of stimulation. Later work with implanted electrodes in unanaesthetised, unrestrained animals has shown that, with some exceptions noted below, behavioural arousal is

accompanied by a similar EEG change whether alerting occurs
naturally or by stimulation of the reticular core. Segundo has
shown that in the latter case alert behaviour can be evoked at

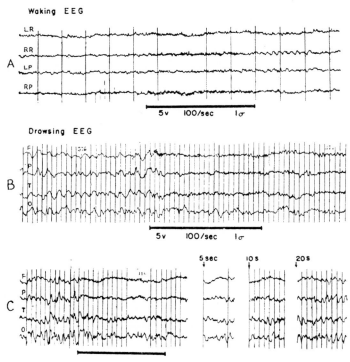

FIG. 120. THE EFFECT ON THE EEG OF THE MONKEY OF
STIMULATING THE BRAIN STEM RETICULAR FORMATION

A: In the alert animal only a slight acceleration of the already fast activity
is detectable.
B: In the drowsing animal the high-voltage slow waves are replaced by
low-voltage fast activity.
C: Sections of records taken 5 sec, 10 sec and 20 sec after the end of
stimulation are given to show the persisting nature of the EEG activation.
The black line beneath each record indicates duration of stimulation.
(From French, Amerongen and Magoun (1952) *Arch. Neurol. Psychiat.*
(*Chic.*), **68,** 577.)

far lower intensities of current than are needed to awake an
animal by direct stimulation of its cortex. In fact generalised
activation by local stimulation of the cortex is apparently
mediated through the reticular formation, the effective cortical

sites being those which, on receiving single shocks give evoked responses in the reticular core, and whose activation has been shown to interfere with ascending reticular impulses (Fig. 121).

The length of the brain stem from which this effect can be elicited extends from the level of the bulb forward through the pons and mesencephalic tegmentum to the lower regions of the thalamus. It thus overlaps at the bulbar level the region from which Magoun and Rhines obtained descending inhibitory

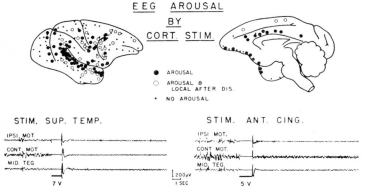

FIG. 121. EEG ACTIVATION IN THE MONKEY BY CORTICAL
STIMULATION

Filled circles show the distribution (on the lateral and medial aspects of the cortex) of sites, stimulation of which evokes generalised fast activity in the cortex and mid-brain tegmentum. Below are examples of responses to stimulation of the superior temporal and the cingulate gyrus. Note that cortical activation is accompanied by reticular activation.

(From Segundo, Naquet and Buser (1955) *J. Neurophysiol.*, **18**, 236.)

effects on motor movement. The fact that the activating effect is more readily obtained by high frequencies than by low suggests that the pathways involve several relays whose many synapses need multiple bombardment and temporal summation before they freely transmit excitatory impulses. This poly-synaptic ascending system is markedly more sensitive to meta-bolic changes and to anaesthesia than are classical sensory pathways.

In their initial experiments Moruzzi and Magoun found the electrocortical effect of reticular stimulation to be not neces-sarily a generalised one, for with just threshold stimulation activation could be restricted to the ipsilateral cortex. Later experiments in monkeys revealed a degree of topographical differentiation in the reticular formation, some sites giving, on stimulation, generalised low-voltage fast activity all over the cortex, others activation in the fronto-parietal regions only. No site was found that would activate the occipital or the temporal cortex solely. From the preparation of multiple serial sections French and Magoun mapped the regions of the brain stem that yielded generalised cortical activation in the anaesthetised monkey (see Fig. 122).

Lindsley and his associates, from serial sections of their experimental lesions, concluded that, provided the central core of the brain stem was intact, section of the medial lemnisci (bearing proprioceptive impulses), the lateral spinothalamic tracts (conveying pain and temperature), or the ventral (carrying touch and pressure) did not affect the animal's vigilance, or its EEG. In contrast, lesions in the central core, sparing the specific sensory pathways, resulted in the animal having the same EEG and behavioural signs of chronic somnolence as were found by Bremer in his *cerveau isolé* preparation (see Fig. 123). Moruzzi and Magoun concluded that loss of vigilance results from the withdrawal of a tonic facilitatory influence of the reticular formation on the cortex. Interruption of the pathways results in coma of considerable duration.

In both sleep and coma, the tonic barrage of ascending impulses necessary for the waking state is missing, so that the tendency of the thalamic nuclei to synchronise their influence on the cortex is released. Recent work from Moruzzi's school has revealed other strong synchronising mechanisms in the lower pons that are also sleep-inducing. The evidence comes from cats in which transections in the mid pons just behind the trigeminal roots produced a low voltage fast type of EEG, whereas transection just rostral to this resulted in an EEG with typical sleep spindles (see Fig. 124). And there are certainly regions in the lower brain stem, slow repetitive stimulation of which evokes a synchronised EEG, as shown for example, in Fig. 125.

It would appear, therefore, that there are strong EEG synchronising and sleep-inducing influences not only in the thalamus but also low in the brain stem. When the latter overwhelm the tonic activity of the reticular formation, sleep ensues.

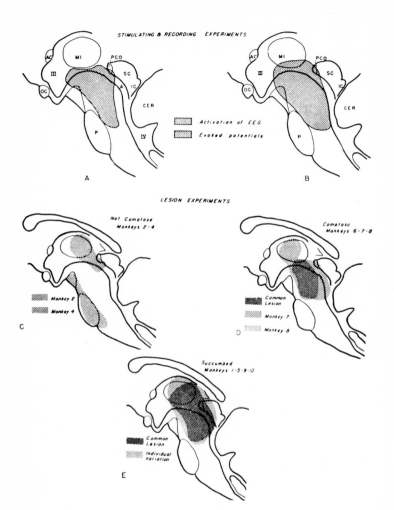

FIG. 122. THE MONKEY'S BRAIN STEM IN MID-SAGITTAL SECTION

Shading in *A* indicates area, stimulation of which causes EEG activation, and in *B* the area from which potentials were recorded in response to afferent stimulation.

The monkeys whose lesions are shown at *C* were not comatose. Lesions mapped in *D* and *E* resulted in coma.

(From French and Magoun (1952) *Arch. Neurol. Psychiat.* (*Chic.*), **68,** 591.)

Arousal of an animal through his own sensory modalities had been the subject of early studies by Ectors, and by Rheinberger and Jasper who established the typical 'activation' pattern of

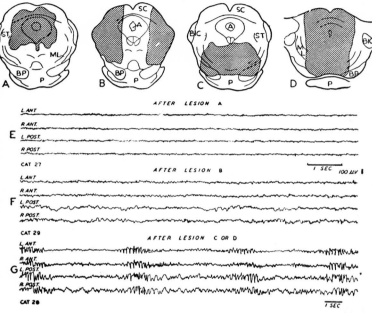

FIG. 123. SCHEMATIC DRAWINGS COMPILED FROM SERIAL SECTIONS SHOWING EXPERIMENTAL LESIONS IN THE BRAIN STEM OF A CAT, WITH (BELOW) RECORDS

Lesion *A*, obliterating the periaqueductal grey, and lesion *B*, sectioning the medial lemniscus, did not abolish EEG activation, as shown by records *E* and *F*. Lesions such as *C* and *D*, both of which include the reticular formation, prevented activation, as seen by the persistent spindling in record *G*.

(From Lindsley, Bowden and Magoun (1949) *Electroenceph. clin. Neurophysiol.*, **1**, 475.)

low-voltage fast activity following natural stimuli. The similarity of this activity to that evoked by reticular stimulation led Magoun to suggest that it might be mediated by fibres or collaterals from the main sensory pathways branching off to synapse on to reticular neurones in the brain stem and, in addition, to some site above the mid-brain. This suggestion, for which there was anatomical evidence from Ramón y Cajal

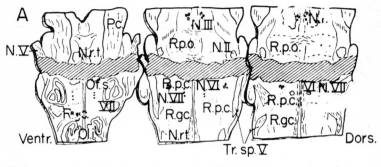

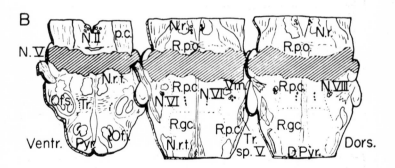

FIG. 124

EEG patterns from right (*F.d.*) and left (*F.s.*) frontal areas following midpontine and rostropontine transection of cat's brain stem. *A*: Midpontine preparation. *B*: Rostropontine. Extent of lesions shown by cross-hatching on drawings of horizontal sections.

(From Batini *et al.* (1959) *Arch. ital. Biol.*, **97**, 1.)

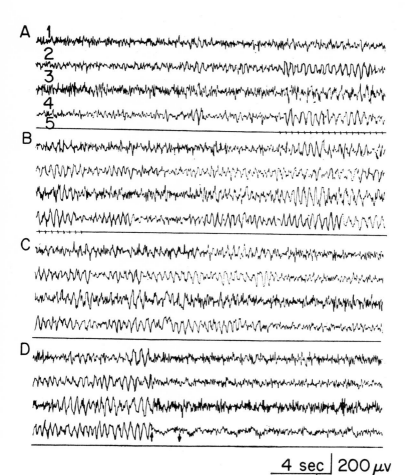

FIG. 125

Development of synchronised EEG activity long outlasting the short train of 10/sec stimulation (at end of *A* and beginning of *B*) of the lower brain stem in the region of the solitary tract. Acoustic stimulation between the arrows in *D* produced an arousal.

(From Magnes, Moruzzi and Pompiano (1961) *Arch. ital. Biol.*, **90**, 33.)

and others (and most recently from Nauta) has received confirmation from electrophysiological studies. According to the
Scheibels, collaterals from the medial lemniscus are not found

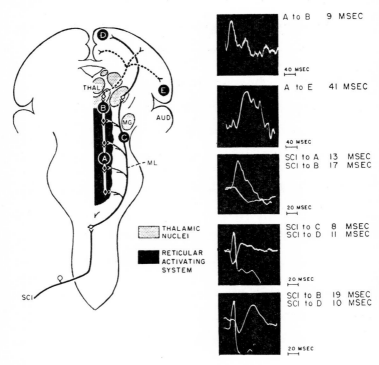

FIG. 126. SCHEMATIC REPRESENTATION OF THE CLASSICAL AFFERENT
PATHWAY TO THE CORTEX

C to *D*: Pathway for impulses evoked by sciatic stimulation. *A* to *B*:
Extralemniscal pathway fed by collaterals from the medial lemniscus (*ML*)
and reaching widely-distributed areas of cortex, including *E*.
On the right are responses evoked by single shocks to the sciatic nerve
and recorded at each of these sites. Note the longer latency of responses
in the extralemniscal system. Negativity recorded upwards.
(From French, Verzeano and Magoun (1953) *Arch. Neurol. Psychiat.*
(*Chic.*), **69**, 519.)

in the caudal medulla but branch off more rostrally at the level
of the ventrobasal complex. In contrast the spinothalamic
tracts have many collaterals ending in the reticular core as well
as in the centre médian of the non-specific thalamus.

Evidence for impulses entering the reticular formation by collaterals from the specific afferent fibres and travelling by midline routes to the cortex has been obtained by recordings within these way stations both by macroelectrode recordings and by single unit studies of reticular neurones. Figure 126, for example, illustrates the responses evoked in the cortex and in the reticular core by sciatic stimulation together with their time-relations. The long latencies are in keeping with a fine fibre or polysynaptic system, and vary with the position of the electrode. If the recording point should happen to lie close to neurones with large fibres the latency would be expected to be shorter than for those with fine fibres or for indirect conduction through a chain of neurones. In all cases, however, the latency at the cortex is longer than that of responses carried by the specific system.

Similar evidence for sensory inflow has been found from the olfactory, optic, trigeminal, auditory, vestibular, vagus, and splanchnic nerves. In fact, the vestibular influence was noted as long ago as 1940 by Gerebtzoff. There is also evidence that sensory stimuli (as well as an artificial, synchronised volley set up by an electrical shock) reach the cortex by this longer route. These responses were not found by earlier workers using animals anaesthetised with pentobarbital, for the ascending reticular system is very vulnerable to barbiturates. In un-anaesthetised, unrestrained animals the responses may be difficult to see because of movement, but techniques for averaging of several responses can reveal them (Fig. 127). Responses from different sensory sources interact, and impulses from one sense modality may attenuate the response from another if the interval between them is short (see Fig. 128).

Lindsley and his co-workers early demonstrated that by certain chronic lesions they could produce a dissociation between the EEG sign of activation and behavioural arousal in cats. Since this dissociation rested on destruction of the reticular core below the thalamus with sparing of all more rostral structures, they proposed that the maintenance of behavioural vigilance depended on excitation of the reticular activating system in the mid-brain although impulses entering above it could evoke a transient EEG change.

The outstanding differences between the afferent inflow to

the cortex that travels through the reticular formation and that of the specific sensory system is that sensory modality is lost. There are two reasons for this, one is that impulses arising from different sense organs often impinge on the same reticular

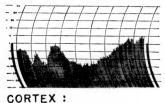

CORTEX :
UNANAESTHETIZED

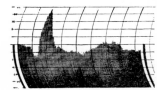

CORTEX : BARBITURATE

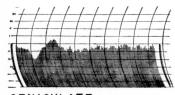

GENICULATE :
UNANAESTHETIZED

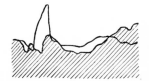

CORTEX : SUPERIMPOSED

FIG. 127. AVERAGED RESPONSES TO A FLASH 10 μSEC IN DURATION
COMPUTED IN 1-MSEC STEPS

Left, above: Cortical response from implanted electrodes in an unanaesthetised cat showing initial surface-positive deflection beginning at 12 msec. Development of surface-negative wave broken into by second surface-positive wave beginning 24 msec after flash.

Left, below: Simultaneous recording from lateral geniculate. Only the primary response is seen, the second having presumably travelled from the reticular formation by an extrathalamic route to the cortex.

Right, above: Pentobarbital anaesthesia induced in the same cat abolishes second response, the principal site of action of the barbiturates being in the reticular formation.

Right, below: The envelopes of the averaged cortical responses, with and without anaesthesia, have been superimposed for contrast. Note longer latency with barbiturate.

neurone (as evidenced by studies with microelectrodes) and the other is that the projections to the cortex from the reticular system are to some extent diffuse and evoke responses in areas other than those specific to the sense organ that initiated the discharge (Fig. 129).

The reticular formation with its wealth of intercommunicating circuits is an important integrating centre not only by virtue of this pooling of sensory inflow, but in addition because cortical and cerebellar efferent volleys also pass into it, as Bremer has frequently stressed. Again the evidence is both anatomical and electrophysiological. Some descending impulses even converge on to the same reticular units as the ascending sensory impulses.

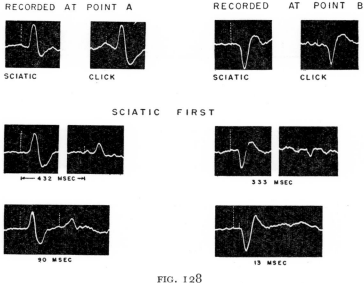

RECORDED AT POINT A   RECORDED AT POINT B

SCIATIC   CLICK   SCIATIC   CLICK

SCIATIC FIRST

|←— 432 MSEC —→| 333 MSEC

90 MSEC   13 MSEC

FIG. 128

Top row: Oscillographic records of potentials evoked at 2 points in the reticular formation of the monkey's brain by single sciatic and auditory stimuli. Point *B* was 2 mm below point *A*.

Lower 6 records: Interaction of the two modalities at different intervals of pairing evidenced by attenuation of second response. Complete occlusion at an interval of 13 msec.

(From French, Verzeano and Magoun (1953) *Arch. Neurol. Psychiat. (Chic.),* **69,** 505.)

This system would therefore seem to have as its function, not the discrimination of one sensory experience from another, but the setting of the stage for conscious perception of the message carried by the specific afferents; in other words the ascending reticular activating system seems to be involved in the alerting of the cortex in what may be the neuronal counterpart to attraction of attention. As Moruzzi has suggested, with the low intensities of sensory stimulation that are to be expected in the physiological animal (in contrast to electrical stimulation) there may be only regional activation of the ascending reticular system resulting in a localised alerting that might form the neurophysiological basis for focused attention.

That an increased level of cortical excitability accompanies the arousal evoked by stimulation of the reticular system has

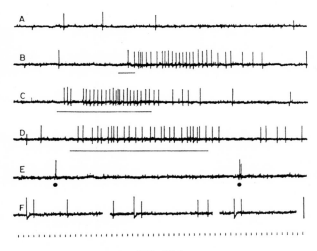

FIG. 129

Convergence of tactile, acoustic and cortical stimuli on to same reticular unit in the pons (cat).
Channel (1), spontaneous activity; (2) tapping ipsilateral forelimb; (3) rubbing back; (4) touching whiskers; (5) acoustic stimulus; (6) electric shocks to sensori-motor cortex. Time line: 10 msec. Vertical marker: 500 μV.
(From Palestini, Rossi and Zanchetti (1957) *Arch. ital. Biol.*, **95,** 97.)

been demonstrated by many workers and for many sense modalities; Bremer and Stoupel, as well as Dumont and Dell, have demonstrated striking facilitation by reticular stimulation of responses evoked by visual, auditory and somatic stimuli (Fig. 130), and Granit has published similar findings (Fig. 131) for unit recordings from the cat's retina evoked by flash stimuli.

In addition, further work has suggested that the reticular formation may play a part as a modulator for the phylogenically older parts of the brain which, as recently emphasised by MacLean, are believed to be concerned with emotion. The

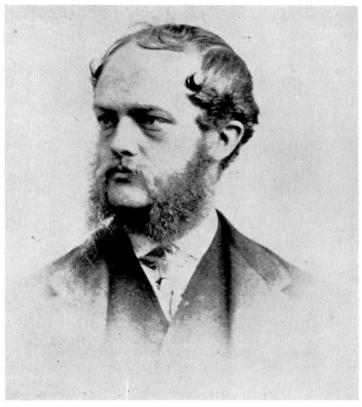

Richard Caton (1842–1926)

The discoverer of the electroencephalogram

'Feeble currents of varying direction pass through the multiplier when electrodes are placed on two points of the external surface, or one electrode on the grey matter, and one on the surface of the skull.'

(Photograph by courtesy of Miss Anne Caton)

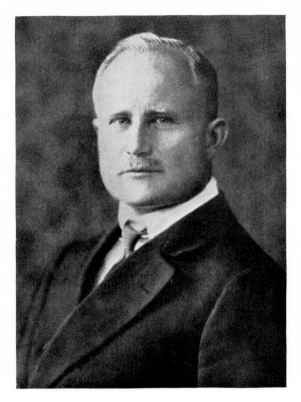

PLATE VIII

Hans Berger (1873–1941)

The first to record the electroencephalogram of man and to apply the technique to clinical problems.

'Ich glaube also in der Tat, das Elektrenkephalogramm des Menschen gefunden und hier zum ersten Male veroffentlicht zu haben.'

(Photograph from Kolle, *Grosse Nervenartzte*. Stuttgart, Thieme. 1956)

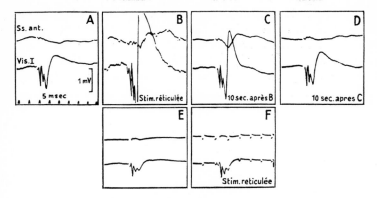

FIG. 130. RESPONSES FROM THE CORTEX OF A CAT TO SHOCK
STIMULATION OF THE OPTIC NERVE

A: Without reticular stimulation. *B*: Facilitation of response of visual cortex (*Vis.* 1) during reticular stimulation. *C*: Facilitation still present but waning 10 sec after end of reticular stimulation. *D*: Return to baseline 10 sec after *C*. *E* and *F*: Facilitation abolished by barbiturate anaesthesia.

(From Bremer and Stoupel (1959) *Arch. int. Physiol.*, **67**, 240.)

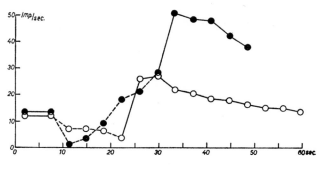

FIG. 131

Number of unit discharges of a cell in the cat's retina. Broken lines: before stimulation of the reticular formation. Solid line, open circles: during stimulation of the reticular formation at 49/sec frequency. Solid line, black dots: during stimulation of 107/sec and at twice the current.

(From Granit (1955) *Receptors and Sensory Perception*. Yale University Press, New Haven.)

257

cortex of the hippocampus in the rabbit has been shown by
Green and Arduini to have a characteristic form of electrical
activity that is the inverse of that seen in the neocortex. In the
alert waking rabbit or in the rabbit aroused by reticular stimulation, the hippocampal discharge consists of regular, synchron-

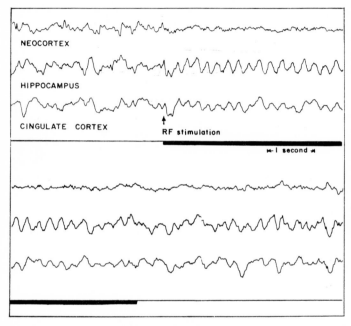

FIG. 132. CONTRASTING EFFECT OF HIGH-FREQUENCY STIMULATION
IN THE RETICULAR FORMATION ON NEOCORTEX, HIPPOCAMPUS AND
CINGULATE CORTEX IN THE UNANAESTHETISED RABBIT IMMOBILISED
WITH FLAXEDIL

Upper and lower records are continuous.

ised waves, usually of 4 to 6 c/s frequency (the so called 'theta'
activity). Simultaneously the neocortex shows fast activity of
low voltage (Fig. 132). This inverse relationship is also evident
on sensory stimulation, as was observed some years ago by Jung.

In the rabbit similar types of responses can be traced in the
relay paths from the hippocampus to the mammillary bodies,
the nucleus anteroventralis of the thalamus and the cingulate
gyrus. In the cat and the monkey with their higher proportion

of neocortex, these contrasting responses of the old brain are more difficult to find and, as yet, have not been seen in man although search has been made in patients in whom hippocampal leads have been implanted for diagnostic and therapeutic reasons.

As indicated above, the ascending system lies in the reticular formation and the tegmentum of the lower brain stem and runs up through subthalamus, dorsal hypothalamus, and ventral medial part of the thalamus. This pathway was found by Magoun and his group using the technique of electrophysiology and ablation, and has since received anatomical confirmation from the work of Nauta. Responses to different modalities of sensory stimuli have been picked up at all these sites and EEG arousal can be evoked by stimulation of them by high frequencies. Fibres from the intralaminar nuclei have been followed to (among other structures) the thalamic reticular nucleus—a nucleus bordering on the internal capsule and surrounding dorsally and laterally the anterior part of the thalamus. This nucleus has been shown by Rose to undergo slow degeneration following rather extensive decortication.

Stimulation of these thalamic regions at high frequencies (300/sec) produces an activation of the cortex similar to that evoked from the lower brain stem. Low frequencies have quite a different effect, as will be described below. This upper portion of the non-specific afferent system, lying in the diencephalon, is known as the thalamic reticular system or the diffuse thalamic projection system. It owes its elucidation principally to the work of Morison and Dempsey, and of Jasper and his associates. There is evidence, however, that the ascending reticular activating system of the brain stem has, in addition, extrathalamic routes to the cortex, for Magoun has found its activating effect to survive destruction of the thalamus. This alternative route passes directly from the subthalamus and hypothalamus into the internal capsule, a pathway that closely parallels that of the Forbes secondary discharge (see page 213).

As might be expected, stimulation of the brain stem produces some circulatory influences that can be detected at the cortex. Ingvar has noted changes in cortical blood flow secondary to EEG activation and both Dell and Rothballer have demonstrated activation of the EEG pattern by the direct action of adrenalin on certain neural elements in the rostral brain stem. Activation mediated humorally is, however, delayed in onset and not immediate as when neurally conducted. In the latter case, only when the stimulus is so weak as to require temporal summation is there any appreciable delay on stimulation in the intact animal. Not all the synapses in the brain stem are adrenergic and some of the apparent discrepancies between behaviour and EEG pattern induced by pharmacological agents (such as atropine and physostigmine) may derive from different levels of adrenergic and cholinergic transmission.

It seems likely that the humoral influence acts as a regulator for the general level of activity of the neural elements in the reticular formation.

THE THALAMIC RETICULAR SYSTEM

In a series of studies on thalamo-cortical relationships by Dempsey and Morison in the 1940s, one of the many important findings that emerged was that slowly repeated stimulation of medial (non-specific) nuclei in the intralaminar regions of the thalamus, at slow rates not far different from that of the animal's own cortical potentials, can bring their rhythms into step and pace them to the exact repetition rate of the stimulus pulse. The pattern of these waves, as well as their distribution, resembles very closely the spindle bursts that dominate the EEG of animals under barbiturate anaesthesia. Work by Evarts and Magoun has, however, shown that they can be evoked in the awake, freely-moving animal by stimulation through electrodes chronically implanted in the medial thalamus. Since these paced, surface-negative responses slowly build up in amplitude during the first few stimuli of a series, Dempsey and Morison named them the *recruiting response* (see Fig. 133). Single shocks to these same subcortical structures trip off trains of waves or 'spindle bursts' in the same widely-distributed cortical areas.

Morison and Dempsey in their original study differentiated between the recruiting response evoked by slow stimulation of non-specific thalamic nuclei, and the *augmenting response* seen on stimulation of an association nucleus. Recruiting responses are of long latency, widely distributed over the cortex, and are predominantly surface-negative. Augmenting responses are of shorter latency, are restricted to the projection area served by the particular nucleus and are diphasic, having an initial surface positivity. This is followed by a slow surface-negative dendritic wave. In both cases the surface-negative component is depressed by simultaneous high-frequency stimulation of the reticular formation. These two types of activity that increase in amplitude on repetition of the stimulus are illustrated in Fig. 133. Their different characteristics have made them useful

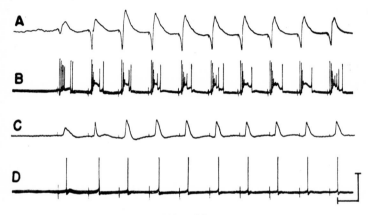

FIG. 133

Augmenting responses (A and B) evoked by stimulation of specific nucleus ventralis lateralis (cat). Recording from cortical surface in A, from inside cortical cell in B. Note short latency and initial surface positivity in A and enhancement of EPSPs in B, as low frequency stimulation proceeds. Recruiting responses (C and D) evoked by low frequency stimulation of non-specific nucleus, centre médian. Recording from cortical surface in C, from inside the cortical cell in D. Note long latency and prominent surface negativity in C and low-amplitude short-duration EPSPs in D. Vertical bar calibration for intracellular potentials = 50 mV.

(From Purpura, Shofer and Musgrave (1964) *J. Neurophysiol.*, **27**, 133.)

signs for the electrophysiologist to use in tracing systems in the living brain.

Greater insight into the neuronal processes underlying the phenomena of augmenting and recruiting responses has come from intracellular recording and more recent understanding of time-characteristics of excitatory and inhibitory postsynaptic potentials. The prominent initial surface positive component that usually distinguishes the waveform of the augmenting from the recruiting response is found to be a short-latency depolarisation of the cortical neurone. This excitatory postsynaptic potential may persist into the surface-negative component or may be interrupted by an inhibitory postsynaptic potential. Recruiting responses are usually accompanied by a slow build-up of EPSPs often with spike discharges, though many varieties of combinations of EPSPs and IPSPs have been found. There does not seem to be a direct correlation between the different phases of the surface recorded responses and the pattern of post-synaptic potentials of any one class of cortical cell. What emerges clearly from Purpura's work is that impulses arriving in (augmenting) afferents from the specific thalamus may make synaptic contact with the same cortical neurones as (recruiting) afferents from the non-specific thalamus. The difference in response lies in the type of postsynaptic potential evoked at their respective points of contact with the postsynaptic membrane.

As originally noted by Morison and Dempsey, recruiting responses can more readily be obtained from the association cortex than from the specific sensory-receiving areas. In parallel with this the anatomical studies of Nauta established connexions between the intralaminar regions and the association nuclei of the thalamus, but failed to find any connexions with the geniculate bodies. Recruitment has also been demonstrated in the caudate nucleus, and a topographical projection from the intralaminar system to the caudate nucleus has been traced anatomically by Droogleever-Fortuyn. The final pathways to the neocortex, however, have yet to be identified anatomically.

Non-specific fibres arriving in the cortex from as yet un-identified sub-cortical structures were found by Ramón y Cajal (see Fig. 114), by Lorente de Nó, and more recently by the Scheibels. It has been proposed that these may form the ana-tomical substrate for the electrophysiologically-demonstrated influence of the thalamic reticular formation on the cortex. These fibres have been found to divide into several parallel paths at entry to the cortex and to give off many collaterals that run parallel to the surface at all layers. Should later work prove these to be indeed the final projections of the thalamic reticular system they would amply provide for a diffuse dissemination of activity, for their collaterals, radiating in the upper five layers of the cortex, are in a position to make axo-dendritic synapsis with the apical dendrites of pyramidal cells. The pyramidal cells receiving their impetus from the specific sensory systems and responsible for outflow from the cortex could thus be modulated in their excitability by depolarisation changes set up in their long dendrites by impulses arriving in non-specific afferents.

In the thalamus the critical points for evoking recruitment by stimulation are found between the level of the mammillary bodies and that of the optic chiasm in the intralaminar cell groups* that lie in the interstices around the specific thalamic nuclei, and in the thalamic reticular nuclei in the external medullary lamina surrounding them. Findings conflict as to whether effective stimulation points are distributed throughout the total length of the thalamic reticular nucleus, but they seem to predominate in its more cephalic extension. Additional sites for evoking recruitment have been found in the nucleus ventralis anterior, in centralis medialis, reuniens and supra-geniculatus. Jasper finds some degree of topographical organi-sation even in this diffuse system, for not only is its influence predominantly ipsilateral, but in addition he finds that the more caudal points influence more prominently the occipital polar cortex and the more cephalic ones the frontal pole. There is undoubtedly considerable interplay through interneurones within the thalamus, for stimulation of any one of the thalamic nuclei from which recruiting responses originate evokes them locally in all others and in the association nuclei of the thala-mus as well, though not in its specific nuclei.

The diffuse effect is independent of the specific thalamic radiations and survives destruction of their nuclei. As men-tioned above, no direct fibre connexions from the intralaminar nuclei to the cortex of the convexity of the hemispheres have yet been traced anatomically, but some have been found to go to the cortex on the medial surface and many to the caudate nucleus and putamen. These fibres emerge from the thalamus and travel in the ventral part of the internal capsule to the corpus striatum, forming a direct thalamostriate connexion.

At the present stage of knowledge of this recruiting system it seems likely that the final terminations in the cortex make axo-dendritic synapsis with cortical neurones, the build-up in amplitude being a summing of the non-refractory synaptic

* The intralaminar groups include the following nuclei: centre médian, parafasciculus, limitans, paracentralis, centralis lateralis.

potentials of the dendrites (see Chapter 9). As will be discussed later in the chapter on electroencephalographic potentials, the latter have all the signs of summed synaptic potentials in dendrites and it is therefore readily understandable that afferent impulses ascending in the diffuse system have a controlling effect on the EEG. Two other electrical signs of dendritic activity that have already been discussed (page 212), the surface negative component of the specific response evoked by sensory stimulation and the sensory after-discharge, are both affected by activity in the diffuse ascending system. To these may be added the augmenting response of Dempsey and Morison, and the surface-negative wave evoked by direct stimulation of the cortical surface (see Chapter 16). The surface-negative components of these responses, like those of the recruiting system, can all be blocked by activation of the ascending reticular system. The clue to the mechanism by which this is mediated may lie in Arduini's demonstration of a generalised steady potential shift towards surface negativity during reticular stimulation, a shift of the background against which discrete dendritic responses may be lost or diminished. An alternative to this hypothesis has been proposed by Purpura who interprets blocking of the surface-negative potentials as an inhibitory action on dendritic activity.

Jasper, whose studies have contributed so much to knowledge of the thalamic reticular system, has proposed a hypothesis regarding its function. According to his suggestion, the diencephalic component of the ascending activating system serves to mediate sudden brief shifts of attention in response to shades of sensory stimulation, whereas the mid-brain reticular system is responsible for maintenance of wakefulness over long periods of time. This suggestion of a differentiation between a phasic and a tonic activation of the cortex comes at a time when the influence of the reticular system in habituation to repeated stimuli and in conditioned learning is of prominent interest.

BIBLIOGRAPHY

Adey, W. R., Segundo, J. P. and Livingston, R. B. (1957) Cortical influences on brain stem conduction. *J. Neurophysiol.*, **20**, 1–16.
Ajmone Marsan, C. (1958) Recruiting response in cortical and subcortical structures. *Arch. ital. Biol.*, **96**, 1–16.

Arduini, A. (1958) 'Enduring potential changes evoked in the cerebral cortex by stimulation of brain stem reticular formation and thalamus.' In *Reticular Formation of the Brain*. Little, Brown, Boston.

Batini, C., Moruzzi, G., Palestini, M., Rossi, G. F. and Zanchetti, A. (1959) Effects of complete pontinetransections on the sleep-wakefulness rhythm; the midpontine pretrigeminal preparation. *Arch. ital. Biol.*, **97**, 1–12.

Bremer, F. (1935) Cerveau isolé et physiologie du sommeil. *C. R. Soc. Biol. (Paris)*, **118**, 1235–1242.

Bremer, F. and Stoupel, N. (1959) Facilitation et inhibition des potentiels evoqués corticaux dans l'eveil cérébral. *Arch. int. Physiol. Biochim.*, **67**, 240–275.

Bremer, F. and Terzuolo, C. (1954) Contributions a l'étude des mécanismes physiologiques du maintien de l'activité vigile du cerveau. Interaction de la formation réticulée et de l'écorce cérébrale dans le processus du réveil. *Arch. int. Physiol.*, **62**, 157–178.

Dell, P., Bonvallet, M. and Hugelin, A. (1954) Tonus sympathique, adrénaline et controle réticulaire de la motricité spinale. *Electroenceph. clin. Neurophysiol.*, **6**, 599–618.

Dempsey, E. W. and Morison, R. S. (1942) Production of rhythmically recurrent cortical potentials after localised thalamic stimulation. *Amer. J. Physiol.*, **135**, 293–300.

Droogleever-Fortuyn, J. and Stefens, R. (1951) On the anatomical relations of the intralaminar and midline cells of the thalamus. *Electroenceph. clin. Neurophysiol.*, **3**, 393–400.

Dumont, S. and Dell, P. (1960) Facilitation réticulaire des mécanismes visuels corticaux. *Electroenceph. clin. Neurophysiol.*, **12**, 769–796.

Evarts, E. V. and Magoun, H. W. (1957) Some characteristics of cortical recruiting responses in unanesthetised cats. *Science*, **125**, 1147–1148.

French, J. D., Van Amerongen, F. K. and Magoun, H. W. (1952) An activating system in the brain stem of the monkey. *Arch. Neurol. Psychiat. (Chic.)*, **68**, 577–590.

French, J. D., Hernández Peón, R. and Livingston, R. B. (1955) Projections from cortex to cephalic brain stem (reticular formation) in monkey. *J. Neurophysiol.*, **18**, 74–95.

French, J. D. and Magoun, H. W. (1952) Effects of chronic lesions in central cephalic brain stem of monkeys. *Arch. Neurol. Psychiat. (Chic.)*, **68**, 591–604.

French, J. D., Verzeano, J. and Magoun, H. W. (1953) An

extra-lemniscal sensory system in the brain. *Arch. Neurol. Psychiat.* (*Chic.*), **69**, 505–518.

Gerebtzoff, M. A. (1940) Recherches sur la projection corticale du labyrinthe. *Arch. int. Physiol.*, **50**, 59–99.

Green, J. D. and Arduini, A. (1954) Hippocampal electrical activity in arousal. *J. Neurophysiol.*, **17**, 533–557.

Hanbery, J., Ajmone Marsan, C. and Dilworth, M. (1954) Pathways of non-specific thalamo-cortical projection system. *Electroenceph. clin. Neurophysiol.*, **6**, 103–118.

Hanbery, J. and Jasper, H. H. (1953) Independence of diffuse thalamocortical projection system shown by specific nuclear destruction. *J. Neurophysiol.*, **16**, 252–271.

Hugelin, A. and Bonvallet, M. (1957) Tonus cortical et contrôle de la facilitation motrice d'origine réticulaire. *J. Physiol.* (*Paris*), **49**, 1171–1200.

Jasper, H. H. (1949) Diffuse projection systems: the integrative action of the thalamic reticular system. *Electroenceph. clin. Neurophysiol.*, **1**, 405–421.

Jasper, H. H. (1954) 'Functional properties of the thalamic reticular system.' In *Brain Mechanisms and Consciousness.* Blackwell, Oxford.

Jasper, H. H. (1958) 'Recent advances in our understanding of ascending activities of the reticular system.' In *Reticular Formation of the Brain.* Little, Brown, Boston.

Jasper, H. H. and Ajmone Marsan, C. (1952) Thalamocortical integrating mechanisms. *Res. Publ. Ass. nerv. ment. Dis.*, **30**, 493–512.

Jung, R. and Kornmüller, A. E. (1938) Eine Methodik der Ableitung lokalisierter Potentialschwankungen aus subcorticalen Hirngebieten. *Arch. Psychiat. Nervenkr.*, **109**, 1–30.

King, E. E., Naquet, R. and Magoun, H. W. (1957) Alterations in somatic afferent transmission through the thalamus by central mechanisms and barbiturates. *J. Pharmacol. exp. Ther.*, **119**, 48–63.

Lindsley, D. B., Bowden, J. W. and Magoun, H. W. (1949) Effect upon the EEG of acute injury to the brain stem activating system. *Electroenceph. clin. Neurophysiol.*, **1**, 475–486.

Lindsley, D. B., Schreiner, L. L., Knowles, W. B. and Magoun, H. W. (1950) Behavioral and EEG changes following chronic brain stem lesions in the cat. *Electroenceph. clin. Neurophysiol.*, **2**, 483–498.

Machne, X., Calma, L. and Magoun, H. W. (1955) Unit activity of central cephalic brain stem in EEG arousal. *J. Neurophysiol.*, **18**, 547–558.

Magoun, H. W. (1944) Bulbar inhibition and facilitation of motor activity. *Science*, **100**, 549–550.

Magoun, H. W. (1950) Caudal and cephalic influences of the brain stem reticular formation. *Physiol. Rev.*, **30**, 459–474.

Magoun, H. W. (1963) *The Waking Brain*, 2nd ed. Charles Thomas, Springfield.

Magoun, H. W. and Rhines, R. (1948) *Spasticity*. Charles Thomas, Springfield.

Morison, R. S. and Dempsey, E. W. (1942) A study of thalamo-cortical relations. *Amer. J. Physiol.*, **135**, 281–292.

Moruzzi, G. (1963) Active processes in the brain stem during sleep. *Harvey Lect.*, **58**, 233–297.

Moruzzi, G. and Magoun, H. W. (1949) Brain stem reticular formation and evolution of the EEG. *Electroenceph. clin. Neurophysiol.*, **1**, 455–473.

Nauta, W. J. H. and Kuypers, H. G. J. M. (1958) 'Some ascending pathways in the brain stem reticular formation.' In *Reticular Formation of the Brain*. Little, Brown, Boston.

Niemer, W. T. and Magoun, H. W. (1947) Reticulo-spinal tracts influencing motor activity. *J. comp. Neurol.*, **87**, 367–379.

O'Leary, J. L. and Coben, L. A. (1958) The reticular core—1957. *Physiol. Rev.*, **38**, 243–276.

Purpura, D. P. (1963) Functional organisation of neurons. *Ann. N. Y. Acad. Sci.*, **109**, 505–534.

Purpura, D. P., Shofer, R. J. and Musgrave, F. S. (1964) Cortical intracellular potentials during augmenting and recruiting responses. II. *J. Neurophysiol.*, **27**, 133–151.

Ramón y Cajal, S. (1909) *Histologie du Système Nerveux de l'Homme et des Vertébrés*. Vol. I. Maloine, Paris.

Rhines, R. and Magoun, H. W. (1946) Brain stem facilitation of cortical motor response. *J. Neurophysiol.*, **9**, 216–229.

Roger, A., Rossi, G. F. and Zirondoli, A. (1956) Le rôle des afférences des nerfs craniens dans le maintien de l'état vigile de la préparation 'encéphale isolé'. *Electroenceph. clin. Neurophysiol.*, **8**, 1–13.

Rose, J. E. (1952) The cortical connections of the reticular complex of the thalamus. *Res. Publ. Ass. nerv. ment. Dis.*, **30**, 454–479.

Rothballer, A. B. (1956) Studies on the adrenaline-sensitive component of the reticular activating system. *Electroenceph. clin. Neurophysiol.*, **8**, 603–621.

Scheibel, M. E. and Scheibel, A. B. (1966) 'Patterns of organisation in specific and non-specific thalamic fields.' In *The Thalamus*. Purpura, D. P. and Yahr, M. D. (Eds). Columbia University Press, New York.

Scheibel, M., Scheibel, A., Mollica, A. and Moruzzi, G. (1955) Convergence and interaction of afferent impulses on single units of reticular formation. *J. Neurophysiol.*, **18**, 309–311.

Segundo, J. P., Arana, R. and French, J. D. (1933) Behavioral arousal by stimulation of the brain in monkey. *J. Neurosurg.*, **12**, 601–613.

Segundo, J. P., Naquet, R. and Buser, P. (1955) Effects of cortical stimulation on electro-cortical activity in monkeys. *J. Neurophysiol.*, **18**, 236–245.

Snider, R. S. and Magoun, H. W. (1949) Facilitation produced by cerebellar stimulation. *J. Neurophysiol.*, **12**, 335–345.

Starzl, T. E., Taylor, C. W. and Magoun, H. W. (1951) Ascending conduction in reticular activating system, with special reference to the diencephalon. *J. Neurophysiol.*, **14**, 461–477.

Starzl, T. E., Taylor, C. W. and Magoun, H. W. (1951) Collateral afferent excitation of the reticular formation of the brain stem. *J. Neurophysiol.*, **14**, 479–496.

Starzl, T. E. and Magoun, H. W. (1951) Organisation of the diffuse thalamic projection system. *J. Neurophysiol.*, **14**, 133–146.

18

The Electroencephalogram of Man

THE recording of the brain potentials of man lagged for many years behind their demonstration in animals, partly because in recording through the skull both electrodes lie at a distance from active brain tissue and the potentials are consequently attenuated. The string galvanometer, which came into general use about 1906, introduced a new era in electrical recording and more confirmations of Caton's original finding were made, including Neminski's demonstration in 1925 that recordings could be made through the intact skull.

The first recordings from the human brain were made by Hans Berger in Jena in 1924 and published by him in 1929. Between that date and 1938 Berger published twenty papers on this subject, nearly all bearing the same title: *Über das Elektrenkephalogramm des Menschen*. It is in the first of these that he makes his historic claim, 'Ich glaube also in der Tat, das Elektrenkephalogramm des Menschen gefunden und hier zum ersten Male veröffentlicht zu haben.' This was, indeed, the first demonstration of brain potentials in man and the first use of the word 'electroencephalogram' to describe them. In these papers he laid the foundation for a great part of our knowledge of electroencephalography. He explored many aspects of the use of the electroencephalogram, including its physiological, neurological, psychiatric and psychological applications. He confirmed Caton's finding, made in animals, that the electrical beats orginate in neuronal tissue, and established that they change with age, with sensory stimuli, and with physico-chemical changes in the body. He was the first to record during a major epileptic seizure in man. That the electrical discharges of the brain were abnormal in experimental epilepsy had been demonstrated in animals more than fifteen years earlier, both by Kaufman in Russia and Cybulski in Poland. Berger was primarily a psychiatrist and was led to search for correlations between electroencephalography and psychiatric observations. Unfortunately he framed a theory before he gathered his data and this coloured the interpretations he made of his findings; the result is that very few of his hypotheses have stood up to the test of time, though his major observations have been abundantly confirmed.

After the date of Berger's first publication many laboratories in many countries took up this work and knowledge of this field grew rapidly. A great deal of information was being gained from animal experiments in such laboratories as Bremer's, Bishop's, and ten Cate's, but many workers went ahead at this time with the study of the human electroencephalogram: Kreindler in Romania, Dietsch and Kornmüller in Germany, Adrian and Walter in England, Baudouin and Fessard in France, and Jasper, Schwab, and the team of Gibbs, Davis and Lennox in America.

All workers were able to confirm the essential claims of Berger's work, and the various centres began to specialise in different problems; Gibbs and Lennox in epilepsy, the Davises in the study of normal subjects, Adrian, Hoagland and Jasper in the basic physiological mechanisms, and Walter in the electroencephalogram in brain lesions. Since these beginnings the spread of interest, observation and experiment has been very great. The historical development since 1936 will emerge as the different aspects of electroencephalography are described.

The growth of electroencephalography has really paralleled that of its instrumentation, for when measured through the skull from electrodes on the unshaven scalp these potentials commonly show a voltage difference between the leads of only about 50 millionths of a volt (50 μV), sometimes more, sometimes less, but rarely, in normal man, do they exceed 200 μV. They are usually, therefore, about 1/10 or less of the magnitude of electrocardiographic potentials. Consequently they need considerable amplification before they can be recorded. The development of the modern thermionic valve made possible an amplification not available to the earlier workers and is responsible for the surge in growth of this field in the last thirty years. The invention of the transistor in 1948 has now replaced electronic circuits in many of the modern electroencephalo-graphs. Instruments have now been designed which take into account the necessity for adequate linearity of response of the recording to the varying voltages led off from the head, and for faithful reproduction of frequencies in a range of from 1 to 500 c/s or more, as well as for direct current recordings. The modern electroencephalographs are shielded in such a way as to avoid radiated interference.

The electrodes used can introduce distortion from extraneous potentials such as those of the skin, bimetallic contacts, and, in the case of chlorided silver electrodes, of photo-electric effects; most electroencephalographs are, however, capacitor-coupled at the input stage, so that these effects become attenuated and they are, in any case, easily recognisable by the experienced worker. As a general rule a relatively non-polarisable electrode (such as silver-silver chloride) is desirable, but many other types of electrode prove roughly adequate for general use. The resistance between any pair of scalp electrodes should prefer-ably be below 3,000 ohms when used with most of the com-mercially-available instruments. There is a variety of tech-niques for recording these potentials in the form of graphs of voltage against time. These may be electromagnetically driven ink-writing oscillographs, thermal or crystal type recorders, cathode-ray oscilloscopes or toposcopes.

In the usual designs of recording instruments the potentials from several pairs of electrodes are led in, each through a differential input stage, and are registered simultaneously, each pair having its independent matched amplifying system and recording unit. Recordings between members of a pair of electrodes may be bipolar, i.e. from two electrodes each of which is over active brain, or so-called 'unipolar', where one of the pair is over active tissue and the other on a far distant relatively inactive point. Such an inactive point cannot be found anywhere on the head, and although the mastoid process, the bridge of the nose and the lobe of ear are frequently used as locations for reference electrodes, they are not truly indifferent and actually contribute potentials from the brain region nearest to which they lie. Many errors of interpretation are unfortu-nately to be found in the EEG literature caused by regarding the earlobe or mastoid process as an 'indifferent' reference, negative spiking from the temporal lobe or temporal muscle being picked up by the reference and being interpreted as 'positive' spikes occurring at a distant scalp electrode.

The fact is that no location on the head is indifferent to the electrical activity inside it and no placement will give a truly indifferent reference. Attempts to use non-cephalic references include the use of an electrode on the skin over the spinous process of the 6th or 7th cervical vertebra. An electrode even farther out on the body is satisfactorily indifferent as regards brain potentials although it may introduce muscle and heart potentials. However, these are not easily confused with true electroencephalographic potentials though they distort the record. Other types of reference leads in common use include a circuit in which two electrodes, one on the neck and one on the chest, have a potentiometer between them for balancing out the electrocardiographic potentials. Yet another brings all the electrodes on the head through appropriate resistors to a common point, in this way giving an average of the brain's potentials against which to measure focal changes under any one exploring electrode. In some circuits the exploring electrode itself is omitted from the average against which it is pitted. As knowledge of the sources of electrical activity within the brain has grown, the use of an average electrode as the reference for unipolar recordings is the method that receives most general acceptance.

Both bipolar and 'unipolar' systems of recording contribute information. The unipolar system, in which is noted the potential difference between each of many scalp electrodes and the relatively indifferent average electrode, allows easier plotting of the electrical field of voltage gradients in a manner consistent with physical theory. That electrode which lies nearest to the focus of activity will show the greatest difference in potential in respect to the average of the other electrodes. The potential difference decreases rapidly as the distance from the source increases. Thus, the maximum height of the pen deflection can be used as a localising sign. It is as though the height above sea-level of every peak in a landscape were being measured.

Bipolar recording on the other hand gives one, as it were, the relative heights of the hills and mountains of the landscape without knowledge of the sea-level. Localisation by this method depends on a comparison of the directions of the pen deflections in the several channels when the electrodes are connected to the inputs in such a way that activity at any one electrode common to two of the channels will cause opposite deflections of the two pens. This method of phase reversal was originally used by Adrian and his co-workers in their search for the source of the alpha rhythm, and was adopted by Walter for the localisation of abnormal waves. In practice, use is made of both bipolar and unipolar methods, especially when localisation of activity is the primary interest.

Other types of electrode have been developed for special purposes, including those designed for insertion into the nasopharynx for sampling activity at the base of the brain, and into the external auditory canal for recording from the lateral aspect of the temporal lobe, and a 'sphenoidal' electrode for recording from the temporal tip. Several types of electrode with appropriate holders have been designed for use in the operating room on the exposed brain for investigation of both cortical and subcortical areas. Electrodes for insertion into deep structures, in which they may remain for some days or weeks, are now being widely used for diagnostic purposes. They have the advantage that the patient may be studied in the unanaesthetised state and in more normal conditions of behaviour and environment than the operating room permits.

In his original paper Berger described the normal electroencephalogram as consisting essentially of the two types of rhythm, first observed by Neminski, which he named the *alpha* and the *beta* bands. Alpha is usually regarded as activity in the frequency range from 8 to 13 c/s, which is prominent in the parieto-occipital regions and disappears with visual attention, and beta as the low-voltage activity between 18 and 30 c/s. To be more exact, the waveform recorded by the electroencephalograph is a complex composed of waves of many frequencies with shifting phase relationships and varying amplitudes. In the great majority of normal records, probably owing to a considerable degree of synchronisation of cell groups, the presenting rhythm generally shows the two frequency bands, originally described by Berger. One of the first recordings from a human subject is reproduced in Fig. 134, which Berger made from his young son; this shows mostly the alpha type of waves.

It has been suggested by several workers that the beta activity may be due to some neuronal groups beating in the second harmonic (i.e. at twice the rate) of the fundamental alpha frequency; accordingly, if such groups were to have greater voltage than those oscillating at alpha frequencies they would dominate the picture, and the tracing would be that of a beta type, whereas if they were of only low amplitude their presence in the tracing would merely be as an asymmetry of the alpha waves which would then appear jagged. In the absence of these faster waves the tracing would appear as a more or less purely sinusoidal alpha rhythm. On the other hand, as the physiological studies detailed in the previous section have

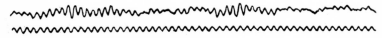

FIG. 134. THE FIRST PUBLISHED ELECTROENCEPHALOGRAM OF A HUMAN BEING

Time signal (lower line): 10 c/s.

(After Berger (1929) *Arch. Psychiat. Nervenkr.*, **87**, 527.)

shown, there is every reason to regard some of the beta rhythms of man as analogous to those fast rhythms of the animal cortex which have been proved to be the result of activity in the ascending reticular system.

In the normal brain when the subject is awake and relaxed, but not alerted, the type of rhythm differs in recordings from different areas. The beta type of rhythm is more commonly found in the frontal part of the brain and the strongest centres of alpha activity are usually located, as Adrian found, in the parieto-occipital regions, although their fields may be spread over other parts of the head as well. However, almost all variations are met with and the above statement applies only to the great majority of normal records. The early hypothesis that the alpha rhythm is generated solely in the occipital poles is no longer so rigidly maintained, the incidence of alpha foci having been demonstrated in other parts of the brain, although they are rare in the frontal regions. The approximate relationship of these major brain areas to certain bony landmarks can be seen in Fig. 135 and a typical recording from a normal subject, when awake and relaxed, is shown in Fig. 136.

In most normal records one frequency stands out more clearly
than all others. This is usually described as the dominant
frequency which, in more exact terms, is defined as the wave-
frequency in c/s which occupies the greater part of the record.
Analysis reveals that more than one frequency in the alpha

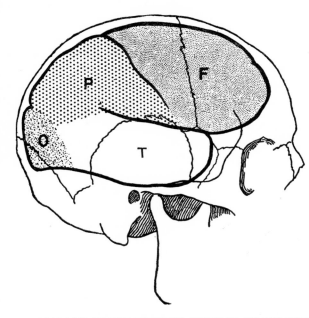

FIG. 135. DIAGRAM OF THE BRAIN TO INDICATE ITS RELATIONSHIP
TO CERTAIN BONY LANDMARKS ON THE SKULL FOR PLACEMENT OF
SCALP ELECTRONS

This shows the gross divisions into occipital (O), parietal (P), temporal
(T) and frontal (F) regions.

band is present in most records. Measurement of large numbers
of records in many laboratories indicates that 95 per cent of
normal adults have, in the occiput, dominant frequencies in
the alpha range, that is, between 8 and 13 c/s. This is also the
average dominant frequency recordable from the parietal lobes
where, however, it may be in some cases a spread by field effect
from the occipital alpha centres. No comparable data have
been published for the frontal lobes, but, as mentioned before,
the rhythms in these regions are very frequently of the fast

beta type, and a simple multiple of the occipital frequency is a common finding. The rhythms of the temporal lobes are in general slower (by 1 or 2 c/s) than those of the occiput.

There are considerable differences in electroencephalograms from person to person, but under standard conditions of rest and relaxation there is little variation in the electroencephalogram

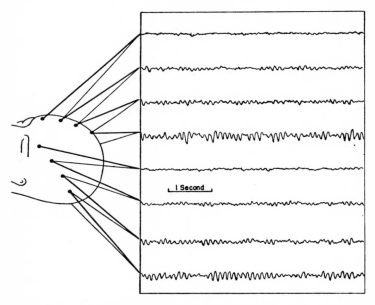

FIG. 136. TYPICAL ELECTROENCEPHALOGRAM OF A NORMAL ADULT
Note predominance of alpha rhythm in the posterior part of the head.

of a normal adult individual, either from hour to hour or over a period of several months. It is this fact which has led workers to feel that the electroencephalogram is a reasonably constant measure of basic physiological significance. Identical twins frequently show superficially similar electroencephalographic patterns, but the evidence is not sufficiently direct to warrant the conclusion that a factor is carried by the genes. More direct information from animal breeding is still lacking.

The frequency characteristics just described for the brain potentials in normal man were originally established by various methods of manual measurement of the tracing. The development of several means of automatic analysis such as those used by Grass, Cohn, Walter, Brazier and Casby, and others, to reveal components hidden to the eye, give a great deal more information.

These early pioneer efforts to quantify the electrical activity of the brain have now been surpassed by the tremendous power of the modern computers for which electroencephalographers have developed many programmes, not only for frequency analysis but for several other aspects of the brain's activity.

In Chapters 16 and 17, the close relationship between thalamic and cortical activity was documented. There is now some evidence that this also holds in man. Records are, of course, unavailable from normal subjects, but in patients with indwelling electrodes implanted for diagnostic and therapeutic purposes, records have been obtained which show the close correlation between thalamic nuclei and their projection cortices, a correlation which does not exist between the neocortex of the convexity and the limbic structures which have no direct projections to it (Fig. 137). These relationships, suggested by visual inspection of the record, have been substantiated by computer correlation analysis.

The electroencephalogram in the awake subject at rest and relaxed is independent of respiration and of heart rate. Overbreathing, on the other hand, with its resultant alkalosis, will eventually break up the normal rhythm of any electroencephalogram. Individuals vary a great deal in the amount of overbreathing they can undertake without affecting their rhythm, but in general most normal adults show no significant change after three minutes of deep breathing, provided their blood sugar level is adequate (that is, not lower than about 130 mg/ 100 cm²). Children have less stable rhythms than adults, and those epileptic patients who have a low threshold to alkalosis also have labile records, a factor which may be used with caution in the diagnosis of this condition.

As mentioned above, rhythmicity of the electrical activity in the parieto-occipital region usually disappears when the eyes are opened, though it tends to return if the eyes are persistently illuminated. This early observation led to a definition of the alpha rhythm as rhythmic activity with a frequency in the range between 8 and 13/sec which disappears when the eyes are opened. Berger's early suggestion was that loss of alpha rhythm results from concentrated attention to the stimulus. In fact, if the subject opens his eyes in a pitch dark room and tries

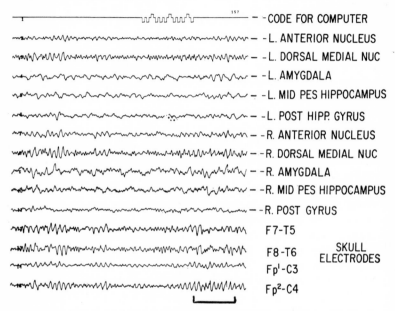

FIG. 137. SIMULTANEOUSLY RECORDED EEGS FROM THALAMIC, LIMBIC AND CORTICAL SITES IN MAN

Note the similarity of activity in thalamus and cortex. Computer analysis reveals a high correlation between the frequencies in these thalamo-cortical regions. The activity in the limbic structures (hippocampus, hippocampal gyrus and amygdala) remains independent. Time line: 1 sec.

very hard to see, the alpha rhythm will be suppressed. Conversely, if in a bright light he wears frosted glasses which blur his vision, the alpha rhythm will persist. It is the attempt to attend to form perception, rather than the light in the eye, which has this effect on the rhythm. The findings are consistent with the clear relationship between electroencephalographic changes and levels of consciousness, in this case an augmentation of consciousness, and they received their explanation when the underlying physiological mechanisms were revealed by

Moruzzi and Magoun's classic work on the influence of the reticular core of the brain stem on electrocortical activity and on vigilance (see Chapter 17).

A more comprehensive definition of the alpha rhythm than that given above would, therefore, be: rhythmic activity with a frequency in the range between 8 and 13/sec which is desynchronised by visual activity and alert attention. This rhythm

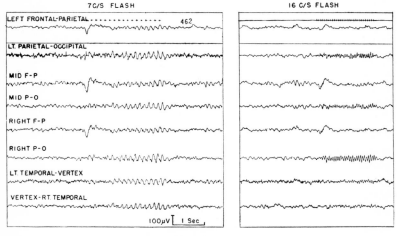

FIG. 138. AN EXAMPLE OF EEG RESPONSES IN A NORMAL SUBJECT TO FLICKERING LIGHT OF TWO DIFFERENT FREQUENCIES

The large slow wave seen in the leads from the front of the head (left F–P, mid F–P, right F–P) are eyeblink potentials at the onset of the flash.

is most commonly found (though not uniquely) in the parieto-occipital regions.

The strong effect of visual stimuli on the synchrony of the beat led Adrian to examine the effect of a rhythmically flickering light. He found, as many workers have since confirmed, that rhythmic potentials can be evoked in the brain which correspond in frequency to that of the flicker within a limited range, from about 6–60 c/s in the normal subject, a wider range in pathological cases (Fig. 138). The two processes, the imposed flicker and the inherent alpha rhythm, compete for the response of the cortical neurones, and it does not seem correct to say that the flicker drives the alpha rhythm, for both can exist together at different frequencies. If the flickering light is diffuse and uniform over the whole visual field, all receptors are equally stimulated at the same moment in time and they consequently respond in unison. This response is in some subjects very clearly seen in the electroencephalogram; in others it is of such low voltage that it is difficult to identify. However, with the added technique of automatic analysis, full descriptions of which appear in the publications of Walter, or by the more modern computer techniques, the evoked response is clearly defined. These techniques are being used in the analysis of flicker rhythms in many widely-distributed laboratories.

One of the details of the response which emerges in the automatic analysis of the flicker response is that with great intensity of light there is not only a response within a given range at the fundamental frequency of the flickering light, but also at twice that frequency (the second harmonic). In man this response at the second harmonic of the flash rate is much more closely localised to the occipital pole than the response at the fundamental frequency, and is less easily disrupted by concentrated mental effort. This finding suggests that the second harmonic may be a response of the primary receiving areas and that the fundamental may be the recruited response of cells whose inherent rhythmicity is closer to the flicker frequency than to the second harmonic.

As a matter of fact in some people the EEG appears to make a differentiation between what one may perhaps call 'vision' and 'gaze'. When the subject is called on to execute certain types of visual task, a typical wave pattern of sharp-peaked 4 to 5 c/s waves appears in the occipital leads. This pattern, first described by Evans in 1952, has been given the name of lambda waves.

In those persons exhibiting this phenomenon, the lambda waves are evoked only when the eyes are open in the light and when the subject is looking at a patterned stimulus which requires searching, scanning movements, for fixation of the gaze immediately blocks the lambda waves. The percentage of people exhibiting lambda waves is so small that it is not surprising that the suggestion has been made that this is an abnormal phenomenon, though its relation to any known disease state has not been established.

Many agents are known to alter the electroencephalogram, those that affect nerve cell metabolism being among the most potent. Among these may be mentioned anoxia, hypoglycaemia and alcohol, all of which result in slow rhythms and eventual suppression of voltage. The effect of drugs, especially the anti-convulsant drugs, has been very widely studied and an extensive bibliography on the subject is being built up. Anaesthetics have varying effects depending on the drug used, but here again the close relationship between electroencephalographic changes and levels of consciousness becomes apparent.

In a previous section the optimal conditions for detecting a response of the cortex to sensory stimulation were shown to be those of deep barbiturate narcosis, the effect of barbiturates being to suppress most of the electroencephalographic potentials before those of the afferent sensory impulses (see page 254). Ether has a different effect, for it blocks activity in the afferent tracts before that in the cortex. Bishop has shown that the action potential of the afferent radiation to the cortex is the last activity to be abolished by ether.

In the human subject the successive stages of slowly induced barbiturate narcosis are very marked, with a close relationship between change in level of consciousness and change in electroencephalographic pattern. In the early stage of thiopental anaesthesia when the subject has not lost consciousness, but is usually, on the other hand, euphoric or confused, the cortical potentials are consistently fast in frequency and generally of high voltage. This type of activity is seen again as the subject emerges from anaesthesia. This change in the electroencephalogram appears first in the leads from the front of the head and persists there longest when the drug wears off. At the moment when the patient loses consciousness the record is immediately dominated by high-voltage slow waves and is strikingly similar to recordings made on patients in a coma or during a faint. If the anaesthesia is deepened a stage may be reached where long isopotential periods are interposed between bursts of irregular waves. This latter stage is not so frequently seen in man as it borders on a very deep level of anaesthesia, but its comparison with the records of Morison and Dempsey at the level used to reveal the spontaneous burst activity in cats is highly suggestive. These successive changes in the electroencephalogram in man during the slow administration of thiopental are illustrated in Fig. 139.

Bremer, in his work on cats, drew attention to the similarity between the electroencephalogram he found in sleeping animals and that found during barbiturate narcosis. The common denominator was revealed by the demonstration of French, Verzeano and Magoun that the principal site of action of the

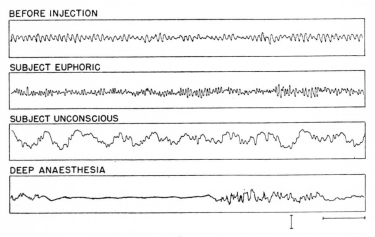

FIG. 139. CHANGES IN THE ELECTROENCEPHALOGRAM OF A HUMAN SUBJECT AT DEEPENING LEVELS OF THIOPENTAL NARCOSIS

Lower right: The horizontal line represents duration of 1 sec; vertical line the deflection for 100 μV. Only samples from the occipital region are shown.

barbiturate drugs is in the reticular formation of the brain stem. In man the change in the electroencephalogram in natural sleep is a profound one.

In the first drowsy stage the usual alpha frequencies are replaced by rather low voltage potentials. The drowsy stage is one in which the subject can very easily be brought back, just by the spoken word, to the fully awake condition. Frequency analysis (Fig. 140) shows that drowsiness has brought with it a shift of the frequencies present from those clustering around 10 c/s to 7 and 8 c/s. Later, in deeper sleep, the frequencies are replaced by slow potential changes of great amplitude and little regularity (see Fig. 141). These are often as long as 1 sec

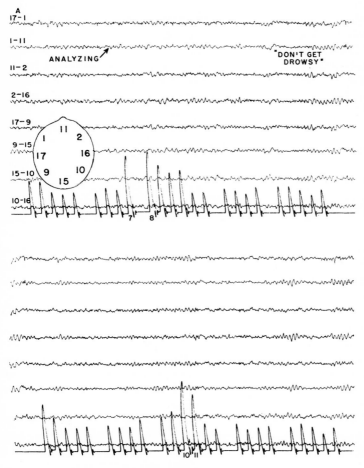

FIG. 140. AROUSAL FROM THE DROWSY STATE

Scalp recording with automatic frequency analysis of the EEG of a normal subject who was drowsy. Note changes of dominant activity from 7 and 8 cycles per second to 10 and 11 when aroused by a verbal command. The second strip is continuous with the first recording.

in duration and are frequently interspersed with trains of faster waves in a frequency range between 14 and 16/sec. These spindles in the records of sleeping man seem analogous to the 'bursts' described by Morison and Dempsey.

This stage usually lasts for only the first one or two hours of sleep and is more rarely seen in the later part of the night when long periods of low amplitude fast activity occur. When recordings are made with amplifiers with suitable time-constants, this activity is found to be riding on slow waves, also of low amplitude. Another feature which differentiates this activity from that of the alert stage is the distribution of the fast frequencies as revealed by computer analysis.

Interest, especially in psychological and psychiatric circles, was stirred when reports began to appear linking dreaming to the stage of sleep when the EEG shows low voltage fast activity, and rapid eye movements are recordable. As rapid eye movements are also seen in sleeping animals this led to the occasional unfortunate description of 'dreaming cats'. However, it has now been demonstrated in many laboratories that dreaming, as reported by human subjects, may often take place during the slow-wave stage of sleep, although this type of mental activity is apparently rather more common when the EEG is in the fast low-voltage stage.

Motor activity other than eye movements and superficial twitches, i.e. discharges from Betz cells, apparently requires a 'waking' cortex, for in man there is usually a return to alpha activity in both thalamus and cortex just before a body movement is made. The slowest components of the sleep records are not equally distributed over the whole head but have two very common foci, one lying precentrally, approximately over Brodmann's area 6 (Fig. 142), and the other farther forward in the frontal region, approximately over area 9. The typical electroencephalographic response to a sensory stimulus during sleep has been described in a previous chapter (see page 218).

There have been some tenuously supported claims that there is a relationship between 'personality' and the alpha rhythm, but the only well-controlled objective study could establish no statistically valid basis for these statements (Henry and Knott). It seems possible that the disturbance of importance in cases that are interpretatively described as 'personality disorders' may

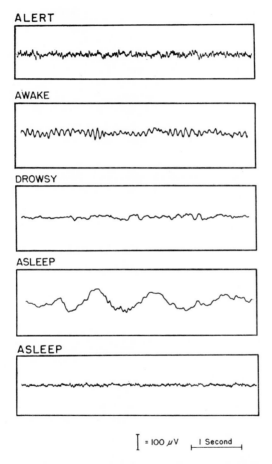

ALERT

AWAKE

DROWSY

ASLEEP

ASLEEP

I = 100 μV |̣ I Second ̣|

FIG. 141. CHANGES IN THE NORMAL ELECTROENCEPHALOGRAM
DURING ALERTNESS, RELAXATION, DROWSINESS AND NOCTURNAL
SLEEP

The delta activity is usually seen in the early part of the night. The
'spindling' superimposed on the slow waves is characteristic of this stage.
As the duration of sleep lengthens these features tend to drop out as shown
in the lowest strip.

be a change in the steering or a re-routing of activity rather than a lesion of structure, and a search for abnormal patterns of distribution may prove more fruitful than has the search for abnormal frequencies as such. If this were so the search for anomalous responses to stimulation might be expected to yield more results than the search for abnormal characteristics in the resting record. That this approach may hold some promise is

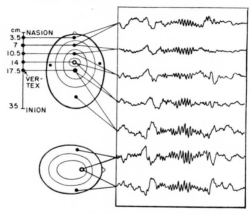

SLEEP:
FOCUS OF SLOW WAVES AND SPINDLES

FIG. 142. SPATIAL DISTRIBUTION OF WAVES IN SLEEP

In contrast to the occipital location of the alpha activity of waking man, the focus of slow waves and the spindles of sleep is found near the vertex.

already suggested by work on the EEG in relation to behaviour, as operationally defined (for example, in controlled experiments on conditional reflexes).

THE ELECTROENCEPHALOGRAM IN NORMAL CHILDREN

The electroencephalogram of the normal child differs from that of the adult. This fact is of significance, not only for the interpretation of records but also, by implication, for the understanding of the brain mechanisms responsible for the electrical activity.

Observation, or measurement by manual methods, fails to

reveal rhythmical electrical activity in the occiput of the normal infant during the first three months of life, although there is evidence of rhythmic electrical activity from the precentral regions even before birth. The remarkable finding is that these rhythms from the precentral cortex are almost of the same order as in the adult (varying from 7 to 13/sec) even before

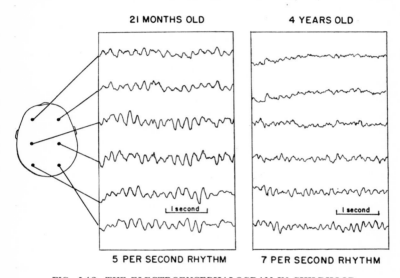

FIG. 143. THE ELECTROENCEPHALOGRAM IN CHILDHOOD

Two samples, taken at different ages to illustrate the change in frequency with increasing age. The chart also illustrates the point that in infancy the dominant rhythm is not restricted to the occiput, as it tends to be later in childhood and in the adult.

birth, whereas those from the occiput, when they first appear at about the fourth month of life, are very slow (3 to 4/sec). The occipital rhythms increase in rate, at first rapidly and then more slowly, until at about 13 years the range of frequencies resembles that of the adult (Fig. 143).

The presence of waves in the sensory-motor area of the infant's brain, before the appearance of any electrical activity in the occiput, parallels to some extent the structural development and maturation of those areas, also the behavioural development of the child. Somatic motor function is evident at birth in the movements and reactions of the child, whereas perception of visual objects, i.e. functioning of cortical visual mechanisms, does not develop fully until the third month.

A quantitative study of a large series of children, many of whom were examined repeatedly over a period of 5–8 years, was made by Henry, whose monograph on this subject establishes standards for normality. The importance of this study is the emphasis it has brought to criteria for the assessment of abnormality in the records of children. In summary, Henry's work defines the characteristics of the normal child's electro-encephalogram as a dominant rhythm slower than the adult's, with slow waves (i.e. slower than 8/sec) always present; these are more prominent in the central areas than they are in the occiput, and decrease as the child's age approaches 13. A chart incorporating Henry's findings is shown in Fig. 144. Walter has used the Greek letter *theta* to designate the band of frequencies between 4 and 7 c/s which in young children's records is a normal feature. An outstanding feature of the records of normal children is their great variability from day to day, in contrast to the comparative stability of the adult's record. It is not surprising that no direct correlation has been found between the electroencephalogram and skeletal maturity, and it is of interest that there is no correlation with the intelligence quotient in normal children.

There have been many reports of abnormal electroencephalograms in children with behaviour disorders. It seems likely that factors such as encephalitis, anoxia at birth, latent epileptic tendencies, and congenital defects of the brain, including failure in completing maturation, may be some of the causes common to both the behavioural and electroencephalographic disorders. The temporal lobe is a suspect region, and again the pattern of distribution of activity may be a clue.

Knott examined the electroencephalograms of a group of normal children with the Grass analyser. The Fourier transforms so obtained showed a relatively high energy peak at 6/sec at one year of age and the gradual emergence of the alpha and beta bands as the age increased. It has been the impression of most workers that occipital alpha frequencies are absent in infants and that the slow waves found in young children gradually accelerate with increasing age until they reach these frequencies. One observer (Dovey) has reported on a group of normal children whose electroencephalograms were analysed by an automatic electronic analyser. From the analysis she concluded that the alpha band of frequencies was present in the occipital regions of all children, even the youngest tested (6 months old), but that it was masked in the unanalysed trace

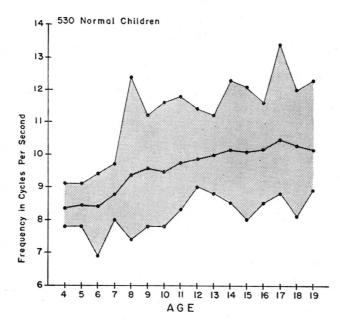

FIG. 144. INCREASE OF MEAN OCCIPITAL ALPHA FREQUENCY IN CHILDREN

The centre curve represents the mean values found at each age, and the grey area the extreme limits encountered in this study of 530 children between the ages of 4 and 19.

(Chart compiled from data published by Henry (1944) *National Research Monograph*, Washington.)

by slower rhythms of higher amplitude. These slower rhythms became less and less prominent as the child's age increased, until at about 10 years of age they were sufficiently insignificant to unmask the alpha band. That this might be the case had been suspected earlier by Smith from observations made without an analyser; he suggested at that time that identification of alpha waves was difficult or impossible when the slower waves were simultaneously present.

BIBLIOGRAPHY

Adrian, E. D. (1944) Brain rhythms. *Nature*, **153,** 360–362.

Adrian, E. D. and Matthews, B. H. C. (1934) Berger rhythm: Potential changes from occipital lobes in man. *Brain*, **57,** 355–385.

Adrian, E. D. and Yamagiwa, K. (1935) The origin of the Berger rhythm. *Brain*, **58,** 323–351.

Baldock, G. R. and Walter, W. G. (1946) A new electronic analyser. *Electron. Engng.*, **18,** 339–345.

Berger, H. (1929) Über das Elektrenkephalogramm des Menschen. *Arch. Psychiat. Nervenkr.*, **87,** 527–570.

Berger, H. (1938) Das Elektrenkephalogramm des Menschen. *Nova Acta Leopoldina.*, **6,** 173–309.

Brazier, M. A. B. (1948) Physiological mechanisms underlying the electrical activity of the brain. *J. Neurol. Neurosurg. Psychiat.*, **11,** 118–133.

Brazier, M. A. B. (1949) The electrical fields at the surface of the head during sleep. *Electroenceph. clin. Neurophysiol.*, **1,** 195–204.

Brazier, M. A. B. (1965) 'The application of computers to electro-encephalography'. In *Computers in Biomedical Research.* Stacy, R. W. and Waxman, B. (Eds) Vol. 1.

Brazier, M. A. B. and Casby, J. U. (1952) Crosscorrelation and autocorrelation studies of electroencephalographic potentials. *Electroenceph. clin. Neurophysiol.*, **4,** 201–211.

Brazier, M. A. B. and Finesinger, J. E. (1944) A study of the occipital cortical potentials in 500 normal adults. *J. clin. Invest.*, **23,** 303–311.

Brazier, M. A. B., Finesinger, J. E. and Schwab, R. S. (1944) Characteristics of the normal electroencephalogram. *J. clin. Invest.*, **23,** 313–317 and 319–329.

Brazier, M. A. B. and Finesinger, J. E. (1945) Action of barbiturates on the cerebral cortex. *Arch. Neurol. Psychiat.*, **53,** 51–58.

Bremer, F. (1937) L'activité cérébrale au cours du sommeil et de la narcose. *Bull. Acad. roy. Méd. Belg.*, **4,** 68–86.

Caton, R. (1875) The electric currents of the brain. *Brit. med. J.*, **ii,** 278.

Davis, H., Davis, P. A., Loomis, A. L., Harvey, E. N. and Hobart, G. (1938) Human brain potentials during the onset of sleep. *J. Neurophysiol.*, **1,** 24–38.

Evans, C. C. (1953) Spontaneous excitation of the visual cortex and association areas—lambda waves. *Electroenceph. clin. Neurophysiol.*, 5, 69–74.

Gibbs, F. A. and Gibbs, E. L. (1952) *Atlas of Electroencephalography.* Addison-Wesley Press, Cambridge, Mass.

Grass, A. M. and Gibbs, F. A. (1938) A Fourier transform of the electroencephalogram. *J. Neurophysiol.*, 1, 521–526.

Henry, C. E. (1944) Electroencephalograms of normal children. Monographs of the Society for Research in Child Development. No. 9. National Research Council, Washington.

Hill, D. and Parr, G. (Eds) (1963) *Electroencephalography: a symposium on its various aspects,* 2nd ed. Macdonald, London.

Jasper, H. H. and Cruikshank, R. M. (1937) Electroencephalography II. Visual stimulation and after-image as effecting the occipital alpha rhythm. *J. gen. Psychol.*, 17, 29–48.

Lindsley, D. B. (1942) Heart and brain potentials of human fetuses in utero. *Amer. J. Psychol.*, 55, 412–416.

Marinesco, G., Sager, O. and Kreindler, A. (1937) Études électroencéphalographiques: le sommeil naturel et le sommeil hypnotique. *Bull. Acad. Méd. (Paris)*, 117, 273–276.

Penfield, W. and Jasper, H. H. (1954) *Epilepsy and Functional Anatomy of the Human Brain.* Little, Brown, Boston.

Prawdicz-Neminski, W. W. (1925) Zur Kenntnis der elektrischen und der Innervationsvorgänge in den funktionellen Elementen und Geweben des tierischen Organismus. Elektrocerebrogramm der Saugetiere. *Pflügers Arch. ges. Physiol.*, 209, 362–382 and 210, 223.

Rémond, A. and Leservre, N. (1965) Distribution topographique et potentiels evoqués visuels occipitaux chez l'homme. *Rev. Neurol.*, 112, 317–320.

Rémond, A. (1961) 'Integrated and topological analysis of the EEG.' In *Computer Techniques in EEG Analysis: Electroencephalography and Clinical Neurophysiology, Supplement* 20. Brazier, M. A. B. (Ed.). Elsevier, Amsterdam.

Sholl, D. A. (1956) *The Organisation of the Cerebral Cortex.* Methuen, London.

Storm van Leeuwen, W. (1961) 'Comparison of EEG data obtained with frequency analysis and with correlation methods.' In *Computer Techniques in EEG Analysis: Electroencephalography and Clinical Neurophysiology, Supplement* 20. Brazier, M. A. B. (Ed.). Elsevier, Amsterdam.

Walter, W. G. (1943) An improved low frequency analyser. *Electron. Engng.*, 16, 236–240.

Walter, W. G. (1936) The location of cerebral tumours by electro-encephalography. *Lancet*, **ii,** 305–308.

Walter, W. G., Dovey, V. J. and Shipton, H. W. (1946) Analysis of the electrical response of the human cortex to photic stimulation. *Nature*, **158,** 540–541.

Walter, W. G. and Shipton, H. W. (1951) A new toposcopic display system. *Electroenceph. clin. Neurophysiol.*, **3,** 281–292.

19

The Abnormal Electroencephalogram
in Man

THE electrical activity of the abnormal nervous system is really
outside the subject matter of this book, but since the rapid
development of electroencephalography in man has been
mainly due to its application to diseases of the brain, a brief
outline will be given here of the chief findings.

Berger, the first to work on human heads, early found that in
the epilepsies the electrical potentials frequently varied from
the normal pattern, a common feature being an excessive discharge as though an unusually large number of neuronal groups
was firing synchronously. Since then very many workers in
different countries have elaborated on his findings and many
different classifications of the abnormalities met with have been
drawn up—too many to detail here. One of the most carefully
developed and well-formulated is that from the Montreal
Neurological Institute. This classification which is widely, but
not universally, accepted forms the main basis for the following
outline; a full account of it will be found in the published
writings of Jasper and Kershman. The descriptions refer to
records taken on the unopened skull and (with one exception)
between seizures.

In the first place a distinction is made between discretely
localised areas of abnormal discharge (Fig. 145) such as suggest
focal damage to the surface of the brain, and more generalised
disturbances presumably projected to the surface from underlying lesions. All in the first category are by definition localised
to a small area of the cortex and the abnormalities are of a
character and time course such as might be expected from
electrical discharges originating not very far below the recording
electrodes; in other words, they are transient potential changes
of fairly short duration which appear spike-like at the usual

recording speeds. They may take the form of isolated *spikes* of about 15 msec in duration occurring at random, or of *sharp waves* (up to 200 msec in duration). When recorded from an electrode over the active area referred to a remote electrode off the head, the spikes are negative at the active electrode. These spikes and sharp waves usually emerge from their background by virtue of their higher voltage. An example of random spikes recorded through the skull, and, later, from the exposed cortex

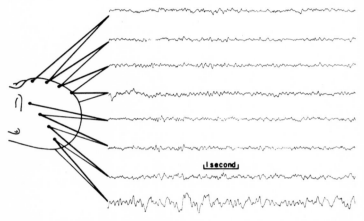

FIG. 145. EEG OF AN ADULT WITH A CLOSED HEAD INJURY

Note abnormal activity localised to the posterior leads over the left hemi-sphere.

of a patient with a cortical scar, are shown in Fig. 146. The increase in voltage and in sharpness of the spike on removal of the skull flap is very marked. The briefest of these spikes, when recorded from the exposed brain, is not less than 15 msec in duration, a time-course more suggestive of a dendritic discharge than of cell or axonal firing. In normal conditions there is no evidence that dendrites do discharge, and this fact, taken together with the observation that spikes are never found in the normal electroencephalogram, lends support to the suggestion that many of the cortical spikes of the epileptic patient may originate as abnormal discharges of the dendrites.

Sometimes the spike activity is seen only as a burst of fairly localised sharper waves against a background of abnormally slow rhythms which may themselves be bilateral. Experience in the operating room in recording from the exposed brain has taught the Montreal group that this last type is frequently the record at the skull of projected activity from a sharp spike focus lying out of reach in a fold of the cortex.

The seizure patterns of epileptic patients whose records fall in this first main category are usually of the focal cortical type.

UNOPENED SKULL   EXPOSED CORTEX

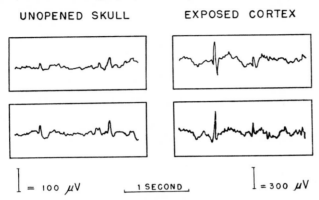

] = 100 μV   1 SECOND   ] = 300 μV

FIG. 146. FOCAL CORTICAL SPIKES IN THE ELECTROENCEPHALOGRAM

Left: From the unopened skull.
Right: From the exposed cortex over the site of a cortical scar (same case). In each of the upper records the exploring electrode is over the focus and the second electrode over another part of the brain (i.e. bipolar recording). In each of the lower records the exploring electrode is over the focus and the second electrode on an inactive point not over the brain (i.e. unipolar recording). Upper and lower recordings are made simultaneously in each case. Note the difference in amplification as shown by the calibration markers below. An upward deflection indicates negativity at the exploring electrode.

In the case of the temporal lobes, however, an empirical relationship has been found between random spike activity localised to these regions and the so-called psychomotor seizures or automatisms. In these cases there is less operative evidence of a superficial lesion. Recent experience has somewhat modified the earlier criteria by which random spike discharges were considered to be the only signs of a local epileptogenic lesion of the cortex. Jasper has now shown that high voltage slow waves may on occasion be of local cortical origin, as also may paroxysmal discharges of rhythmic form.

The second main category includes records of activity at the surface apparently projected from subcortical lesions; these abnormalities are in sharp distinction to those just described, in that instead of being discretely localised in one hemisphere of the brain they are distributed not only bilaterally, but may be synchronous in homologous areas of the hemispheres. They are usually of high voltage. Of these, one form is the *spike and wave*, a type of abnormal activity first described by Gibbs,

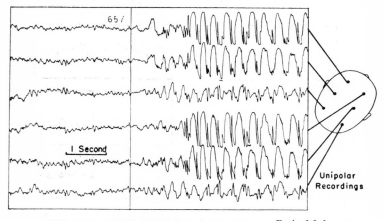

FIG. 147. AN EXAMPLE OF THE ONSET OF *Petit Mal*

Note the bilateral distribution of spike and wave complexes predominating in the frontal regions.

Davis and Lennox, workers who have made very great contributions to this branch of electroencephalography. These spike and wave discharges have usually a regular rhythm of approximately 3 or 3½/sec but they may occur in irregular bursts; they are almost invariably of high amplitude and usually are most marked in the midfrontal region of the head; they are almost always bilaterally synchronous (the exception is the rare traumatic case which shows a localised spike and wave discharge). A typical example is shown in Fig. 147. Unlike the other types of abnormality described here, the rhythmic spike and wave discharges are usually accompanied by a clinical seizure of the *petit mal* type, although this may be very brief. The bilateral synchrony of these spike and wave rhythms and of 3/sec waves appearing without a spike component is certainly suggestive of conducted disturbances from a deep midline trigger zone. There is some experimental work with animals which supports this hypothesis (Morison, Finley and Lothrop; Jasper and Fortuyn), and indicates a diencephalic pacemaker for these discharges.

Other types of generalised abnormality in this second category are bilaterally synchronous bursts of slow waves (3–6/sec) or of fast waves (up to 30/sec), all usually of high amplitude. All the abnormalities described in this second main category are commonly found in cases of the so-called idiopathic type of epilepsy which is usually regarded as congenital or hereditary, since no cause for its having been acquired is known. Abnormalities are commonly found in the records of close relatives of epileptic patients. Approximately two-thirds of these patients have some abnormality in their records between seizures. The waveforms in this category are not specifically related to the clinical seizure patterns and cannot be used to differentiate accurately between the symptom forms.

Less well-defined abnormal wave patterns sometimes seen in the records of epileptic patients include irregularly occurring slow waves, often mixed with sharp waves. However, when these slow waves appear at all continuously they may indicate a lesion, for these are the waves which are found in tissues bordering tumours of the brain, as first described by Walter and named by him *delta* waves. He applied this name to waves slower than 5/sec, a common frequency for them being 2–3/sec.

Finally, epileptic patients may have electroencephalograms which are diffusely abnormal, conforming to neither of the two main categories just outlined. There may be no well-defined single abnormality but many mixed irregularities with, perhaps, even more than one focus. A record of this kind arouses suspicions of diffuse cortical disease or atrophy, but no one-to-one correlation can be made with the clinical picture. Most correlations between the electroencephalogram and the clinical state are still only empirically-established relationships (Fig. 148).

Many methods are used for bringing out electroencephalographic abnormalities for the purpose of diagnosis and possible localisation. The most common of these is for the patient to overbreathe, as the resultant alkalosis increases in some cases both the amplitude and incidence of abnormal discharges, more especially the bilaterally synchronous 3/sec waves and the spikes and waves of non-focal character. Another method used in many laboratories is to recruit the latent rhythm by rhythmic photic stimulation of appropriate frequency. Any latent tendency to abnormal activity may be augmented into a discharge of diagnostic significance and may even precipitate a seizure (Fig. 149). Cardiazol (metrazol) injected intravenously is given by some to evoke the focal type of spike or sharp wave, also

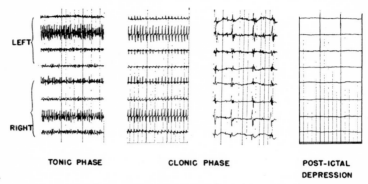

TONIC PHASE   CLONIC PHASE   POST-ICTAL
                                           DEPRESSION

FIG. 148. PROGRESSION OF A *Grand Mal* SEIZURE

EEG examples, each 3 seconds in duration, taken during and after a major convulsion as it passed from the tonic to the clonic phase. After such a seizure the EEG may remain depressed for many minutes.

focal slow waves. An effective type of activation is a combination of small doses of cardiazol with photic stimulation which elicits diencephalic signs at a threshold below the convulsive one. Sleep, either natural or induced by sedatives, has been claimed to be effective in eliciting abnormal discharges in some epileptic patients, particularly those with disorders of the temporal lobe. The electroencephalograms of young children are very unstable and may become grossly disturbed with very little overbreathing so that this method of intensifying abnormal components is less valuable for detecting epileptic tendencies among the younger age groups than among adults. The value of overbreathing for differential diagnosis is also dubious in subjects over the age of 60.

It should, perhaps, be remarked that a small number of

patients with clinical seizures have normal electroencephalograms as recorded from the scalp and, conversely, a few people with no known seizures have electroencephalograms with some of the abnormal features described above. These aberrant cases are too few to detract seriously from the usefulness of the electroencephalogram in the differential diagnosis of epilepsy from that of hysteria or of syncopal conditions (between attacks).

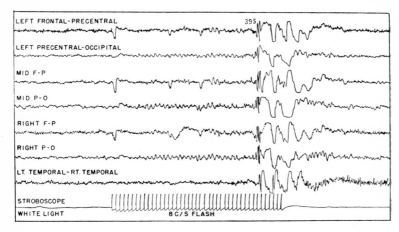

FIG. 149. AN EXAMPLE OF AN ABNORMAL EEG RESPONSE TO FLICKERING LIGHT IN A PHOTOSENSITIVE EPILEPTIC PATIENT

The large slow wave seen in the leads from the front of the head at the onset of light (left *F–P*, mid *F–P* and right *F–P*) are eyeblink potentials.
(From Brazier (1955) *Epilepsia* (*Boston*), **4,** 9.)

Techniques have been developed for implanting electrodes in deep structures within the brain and for leaving them there so that recordings may be made for some days during which the patient may experience one of his typical seizures. Studies of this kind have revealed that episodes of high-voltage paroxysmal discharge may accompany these clinical attacks, but if in regions that have no projections to the cortex of the convexity, the seizure discharges may not reach the scalp electrodes. This is doubtless one of the reasons that normal scalp recordings are sometimes obtained in patients known to have epilepsy (see Fig. 150).

A striking abnormality in the electroencephalogram which

has been found to have an empirical relationship with the presence of a brain tumour is the occurrence of slow potentials having no regular rhythm but usually of high amplitude. These slow potentials, which are sometimes a quarter of a second or longer in duration, are those which were originally named

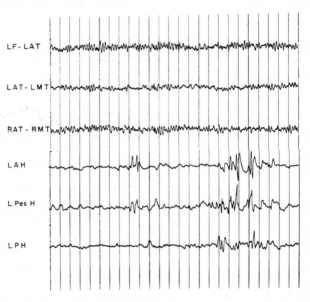

FIG. 150. FAILURE OF SCALP RECORDINGS TO DETECT ABNORMAL
DISCHARGES IN THE HIPPOCAMPUS OF MAN

In the three lowest traces the recordings are from electrodes implanted stereotactically in three sites in the left hippocampus of a patient with temporal lobe epilepsy. The two top traces are from the skull over the convexity of the ipsilateral temporal lobe in frontal (*LF*), anterior (*LAT*) and mid (*LMT*) locations. Trace *RAT–RMT* is from the skull over the contralateral temporal lobe. Length of sample: 5 seconds.

delta waves by Walter for convenience of terminology. Tumour tissue is electrically inactive but a space-occupying neoplasm by pressure evokes abnormal potentials in the brain tissue surrounding it, and may thus be localised by the focus of delta waves it arouses. When the tumour is hemispheric but not very close to the surface the disturbance it creates in the recording from the scalp may take the form of a disruption of the rhythm with the appearance of slow waves, but without the

clearly-defined delta trains usually recordable from tissue more
closely adjacent to the neoplasm (see for example, Fig. 151).
Lesions of the brain stem, however, causing the patient to be
comatose, are usually associated with slow waves appearing
bilaterally at the cortex, similar to those induced by French
and Magoun by experimental lesions of the reticular core in

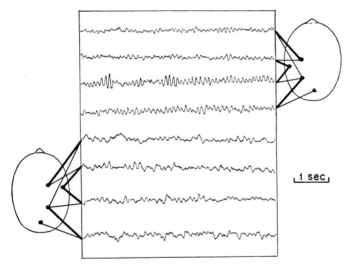

FIG. 151. ELECTROENCEPHALOGRAM IN A CASE OF RIGHT-SIDED
TUMOUR

Excerpt from the EEG of a patient with a tumour in the posterior parieto-
temporal region of the right hemisphere. Note the contrast between the
rhythmic quality of the recording from the normal side with the irregu-
larity and slower waves on the side of the tumour. For clarity, electrodes
on other parts of the head have been omitted from the diagrams.

monkeys (see page 247). Some form of abnormality is found in
about 90 per cent of the records of patients with brain tumours.
    Other diseases of the brain in which delta waves are some-
times found include encephalitic cases, acute vascular accidents
and cortical atrophy; in these cases the abnormal potentials
are less commonly focal in their distribution and seem to be
associated with diffuse cortical destruction. However, where
the cell destruction is itself restricted to a discrete area, the
electrical abnormalities are also likely to be localised.
    A single electroencephalographic test can yield data which

help to locate, but not differentiate between, brain injury, infection, tumour or vascular accident; any of these cases may have epileptic fits which are a sign of cerebral abnormality just as is the electroencephalographic disturbance. Serial tests may, however, give information as to degree and direction of change with the passage of time which can be useful in making a differential diagnosis. For example, the abnormalities tend to lessen with time after a vascular accident, but to increase with an expanding lesion. In head injuries serial tests are usually of great value in helping to determine the amount of damage; the degree of abnormality in the record correlates closely with the severity of the injury. A small percentage of these cases may develop a subdural haematoma and although the electro-encephalogram is not invariably abnormal when recorded from the unopened skull over a subdural haematoma, in the majority of cases some differences can be detected between the recording from the normal hemisphere and that from the side with the clot.

The few examples outlined here of electroencephalographic abnormalities associated with diseased or damaged states of the brain, serve to illustrate the point that the electrical disturbances themselves cannot be classified into types indicating specific disease. With the possible exception of the spike-and-wave discharge which accompanies a clinical seizure in the *petit mal* type of epilepsy, the electrical patterns do not in themselves represent disease entities; they are signals of neuronal dysfunc-tion, and as such may, when knowledge grows, contribute as much to our understanding of the state of functioning nervous tissue as the microscope has contributed to our knowledge of its inert structure.

The development from the concept of the electroencephalo-gram as primarily an aid in assessing the normality of the resting, 'inactive' brain, to a dynamic formulation of it as an indicator of the brain in action, has, with its emphasis on function rather than on morphology, suggested a wider applica-tion of the EEG to the study of behaviour, and it is along these lines that much of the modern work is being directed.

Progressing from the study of the structural design of nervous interconnexion to the dynamics of nervous intercommunica-tion, and to the search for the signals which by their timing and their grouping produce order in place of randomness, integration in place of scatter, our most promising approach is through the study of the electrical activity of the nervous system.

BIBLIOGRAPHY

Ajmone Marsan, C. and Ralston, B. L. (1957) *The Epileptic Seizure.* Thomas, Springfield.

Berger, H. (1929) Über das Elektrenkephalogramm des Menschen. *Arch. Psychiat. Nervenkr.*, **87**, 527–570.

Berger, H. (1932) Über das Elektrenkephalogramm des Menschen. *Arch. Psychiat. Nervenkr.*, **98**, 231–254.

Berger, H. (1934) Über das Elektrenkephalogramm des Menschen. *Arch. Psychiat. Nervenkr.*, **102**, 538–557.

Brazier, M. A. B. (1955) Neuronal structure, brain potentials and epileptic discharge. *Epilepsia.* (*Amst.*), **4**, 9–18.

Brazier, M. A. B. (1958) The developments of concepts relating to the electrical activity of the brain. *J. nerv. ment. Dis.*, **126**, 303–321.

Cobb, W. A. (1944) The electroencephalographic localisation of intracranial neoplasms. *J. Neurol. Neurosurg. Psychiat.*, **7**, 96–102.

Droogleever-Fortuyn, J. (1957) On the pathophysiology of petit mal. *Proc. 1st Internat. Cong. Neurol. Sci.*, 259–271.

Fischgold, H. and Bounes, G. (1946) Exploration électroencéphalographique des états comateux. *Sem. Hôp. Paris*, **22**, 1245–1247.

Fischgold, H. and Mathis, P. (Eds) (1959) *Obnubilations, Comas et Stupeurs.* Masson, Paris.

Foerster, O. and Altenburger, H. (1935) Elektrobiologische Vorgänge an der menschlichen Hirnrinde. *Dtsch. Z. Nervenheilk.*, **135**, 277–288.

Gastaut, H. (1954) *The Epilepsies: Electroclinical Correlations.* Translated by M. A. B. Brazier. Thomas, Springfield.

Gibbs, E. L. and Gibbs, F. A. (1947) Diagnostic and localising value of electroencephalographic studies in sleep. *Res. Publ. Ass. nerv. ment. Dis.*, **26**, 366–376.

Gibbs, F. A., Davis, H. and Lennox, W. G. (1935) The electroencephalograms in epilepsy and in impaired states of consciousness. *Arch. Neurol. Psychiat.* (*Chic.*), **34**, 1133–1148.

Jasper, H. (1950) Electrocorticograms in man. *Electroenceph. clin. Neurophysiol.*, Suppl. 2, 16–29.

Jasper, H. H. and Fortuyn, J. D. (1947) Experimental studies on the functional anatomy of petit mal epilepsy. *Res. Publ. Ass. nerv. ment. Dis.*, **26**, 272–298.

Jasper, H. H. and Kershman, J. (1941) Electroencephalographic classification of the epilepsies. *Arch. Neurol. Psychiat.*, **45**, 903–943.

Jasper, H. H. and Kershman, J. (1950) Classification of the EEG in epilepsy. *Electroenceph. clin. Neurophysiol.*, Suppl. 2, 124–131.

Kaufman, I. C., Marshall, C. and Walker, A. E. (1947) Metrazol activated electroencephalography. *Res. Publ. Ass. nerv. ment. Dis.*, **26**, 476–486.

Magnus, O., Storm van Leeuwen, W. and Cobb, W. A. (Eds) (1961) *Electroencephalography and Cerebral Tumours: Electroencephalography and Clinical Neurophysiology, Supplement* 20. Elsevier, Amsterdam.

Morison, R. S., Finley, K. H. and Lothrop, G. N. (1952) Influence of basal forebrain areas on the electrocorticogram. *Amer. J. Physiol.*, **4**, 265–270.

Penfield, W. and Jasper, H. H. (1954) *Epilepsy and Functional Anatomy of the Human Brain.* Little, Brown, Boston.

Rademecker, J. (Ed.) (1956) *Systématique et Electroencéphalographie des Encéphalités et Encéphalopathies: Electroencephalography and Clinical Neurophysiology, Supplement* 5. Masson, Paris.

Ramey, E. R. and O'Doherty, D. S. (Eds) (1960) *Electrical Studies of the Unanaesthetised Brain.* Hoeber, New York.

Rémond, A. (1952) Photo-metrazol activation. *Electroenceph. clin. Neurophysiol.*, **4**, 265–270.

Schwab, R. S. (1951) *Electroencephalography in Clinical Practice.* Saunders, Phila.

Walter, W. G. (1936) The location of cerebral tumours by electro-encephalography. *Lancet*, **ii**, 305–308.

Walter, W. G. (1950) The principles and methods of location. *Electroenceph. clin. Neurophysiol.*, Suppl. 2, 9–15.

Index

In this index the numbers of the pages on which references appear in the text are printed in ordinary type. Pages giving specially detailed description of a subject are in bold type. Those that refer to illustrations are in italics, and those that refer to authors' names in the bibliographies are enclosed in parentheses.

SUBJECT INDEX

AUTHORS INDEX